Diagnosis

in

Traditional Chinese Medicine

Ping Chen

Complementary Medicine Press
Taos, New Mexico   2004

Diagnosis in Traditional Chinese Medicine
Ping Chen
ISBN 0-9673034-5-1
Copyright ©2004 Ping Chen

Library of Congress Cataloging-in-Publication Data

Chen, Ping, 1953-
  Diagnosis in traditional Chinese medicine / Ping Chen.
     p. ; cm.
  Includes bibliographical references and index.
  ISBN 0-9673034-5-1 (alk. paper)
  1. Diagnosis. 2. Medicine, Chinese.
  [DNLM: 1. Diagnosis. 2. Medicine, Chinese Traditional. WB 50.1 C518a
2004a] I. Title.
  RC71.C55455 2004
  616.07'5--dc22

                              2004004360

Published by Complementary Medicine Press
202 Bendix Drive
Taos, New Mexico 87571

Distributed by
Redwing Book Company, Taos NM
www.redwingbooks.com

Table of Contents

List of Tables and Figures

Council of Oriental Medical Publishers
Designation

This is an original English language work written as a textbook for the author's English-speaking students. A description of the governing terminology and translation method may be found in the glossary.

Foreword

Diagnostics is an important component of traditional Chinese medicine (TCM), serving as the bridge between TCM theory and clinical practice. It includes not only diagnostic techniques, but also the theory and clinical application of pattern identification, which is regarded as the most significant aspect of TCM.

The material for this book comes from many years of teaching TCM diagnostics to both Chinese medical students and university-level Western medical students. I created this book to provide my students with a more complete view of TCM diagnostics practice than has been available in English. I organized my course notes as tables because my English-speaking TCM students found the constant repetition of the main instructional categories (etiology, pathogenesis, and manifestation) confusing when repeated over and over again as narrative prose.

This book consists of two parts. Part One systematically introduces the four diagnostic methods that are unique to TCM, with special emphasis on tongue inspection and pulse examination, the most important diagnostic methods. Part Two discusses the theory and clinical application of the different systems of pattern identification.

The text is arranged into thirteen chapters. Chapter I introduces the main points in the development of TCM diagnostics. Chapters II-V examine the four diagnostic methods: inspection, auscultation and olfaction, interrogation, and palpation and pulse examination. The chapter on interrogation includes symptom patterns, given in the form of tables that list the characteristics of each symptom or sign, along with its pathogenesis and clinical pattern. Reading these chapters will provide a clearer understanding of the methods leading to clinically accurate pattern identification. Chapters VI-XII explain the seven types of pattern identification. They are:

- Pattern identification according to the eight principles
- Pattern identification according to pathogenic factors
- Pattern identification according to qi and blood
- Pattern identification according to the internal organs
- Pattern identification according to the six channels
- Pattern identification according to wei, qi, ying, and blood
- Pattern identification according to upper, middle, and lower burner.

Of these seven, pattern identification in light of organ theory is considered the most important. Included in the explanation for each type of pattern identification are the various manifestations with which a pattern may present; the main manifestations by which a pattern may be identified; an analysis of the etiology and pathogenesis for each symptom or sign of a pattern; and differential diagnosis—for example, those manifestations which help to differentiate one pattern from another. Each pattern is introduced in the order of the main manifestations, common pathogenesis, and systematic pathogenesis. In order to clearly demonstrate the complete philosophic thinking in pattern identification, each pattern is shown in the form of tables. A series of case histories is included in Chapter Thirteen. By comparing these histories with the diagnostic methods of pattern identification introduced in the text, those readers whose goal is to put into practice their knowledge of TCM pattern identification can follow the progression of the philosophic thinking.

Ping Chen, DOM, OMD, MD (PRC)

New Mexico, U.S.A.

CHAPTER ONE

General Introduction

I. Important Milestones in the Development of TCM Diagnostics

During different historical periods in the development of traditional Chinese medicine, many well-known physicians made great contributions to diagnostics. Their names, the era during which they lived, leading works, and their significance in the development of TCM diagnostics are shown in Table 1.1.

II. Clarification of Some TCM Terms

1. Disease

In TCM theory, a disease is a specific process of life. It refers to the result of the interaction of pathogenic factors (known as evil qi) and body resistance (known as vital qi) finally causing the **breakdown** of the balance **between yin and yang**.

The action of pathogenic factors on the body is a result of both organic and functional **impairment**. The body may react to these pathogenic factors in two ways. One is to call up vital qi to **expel** invading pathogens; the other is to call up vital qi to **restore** the impaired functions. Furthermore, as specific life processes, breakdown/impairment and expelling/restoration are always dynamic. Their progression is determined by the dynamic interaction between pathogenic factors and bodily resistance.

2. Manifestation

A manifestation refers to the external display of an internal pathogenic development. It includes both **symptoms** and **signs**. A manifestation serves as the main evidence for pattern identification.

A symptom refers to the **subjective abnormal sensations** felt by the patient, for example, pain, distension, numbness, and etc.

A sign refers to the **objective abnormal display**, which, upon examination, indicates a disease, for example, pale face, skin rashes, or rapid pulse.

3. Pattern

A pattern refers to the highly **pathogenic condensation** of a certain stage of a disease. It implies a group of **manifestations** at a certain pathogenic stage. Moreover, it provides the **perspective for treatment**.

Table 1.1 Important Milestones of TCM Diagnostics

Name	Dynasty	Representative works	Significance
Anon.	Warring States (445–221 B.C.E.)	*Nei Jing (Classic of Internal Medicine)*	Foundations of TCM diagnostics
Chunyu Yi	Western Han (206 B.C.–24 C.E.)	*Er Shi Wu Bing An (Twenty-five Cases)*	First written record of case histories
Zhang Zhong-jing	Eastern Han (24-220 C.E.)	*Shang Han Za Bing Lun (On Cold Damage and Miscellane-ous Diseases)*	Initiated pattern identification according to the six channels
		Jin Kui Yao Lue (Essential Prescriptions of the Golden Coffer)	Initiated pattern identification according to the internal organs
Wang Shuhe	Western Jin (265-316 C.E.)	*Mai Jing (Pulse Classic)*	Earliest monograph on pulse examination
Chao Yuan-fang	Sui (581-618 C.E.)	*Zhu Bing Yuan Hou Lun (Origins and Symptoms of Diseases)*	Earliest monograph on diagnosis based on etiology, pathogenesis, and pattern identification
Sun Simiao	Tang (618-907 C.E.)	*Bei Ji Qian Jin Yao Fang (Thousand Gold Pieces Prescriptions for Every Emergency)*	Perfected comprehensive application of four diagnostic methods and pattern identification
Du Qingbi	Yuan (1271-1368 C.E.)	*Ao Shi Shang Han Jin Jing Lu (Ao's Records of the Golden Mirror of Febrile Diseases)*	Earliest monograph on tongue inspection
Zhang Jingyue	Ming (1368-1644 C.E.)	*Jing Yue Quan Shu (Complete Works of Zhang Jingyue)*	Treatment according to pattern identification synthesized into a complete and independent theoretical system
		Shi Wen (Ten Questions/Ten Aspects to Interrogate in Verse)	Perfected interrogation
Han Feixia		*Han Shi Yi Tong (Han's Comprehensive Medical Views)*	Perfected written case histories
Li Shizhen		*Bin Hu Mai Jue (Pulse Studies of Bin Hu)*	Popularized pulse studies
Ye Tianshi	Qing (1644-1911 C.E.)	*Wen Re Lun (Treatise on Epidemic Febrile Diseases)*	Initiated pattern identification according to wei, qi, ying, and xue
Wu Jutong		*Wen Bing Tiao Bian (Treatise on Pattern Identification and Treatment of Epidemic Febrile Diseases)*	Initiated pattern identification according to the three burners

4. TCM Diagnostics

TCM diagnostics refers to the study of a disease according to TCM theories and therapies, followed by the assignment of a pattern type to the disease. A diagnosis refers to the judgment from a physician as to the **state of the constitution,** as well as the **name of the disease** and its **pattern types.**

III. Essential Ideas for Studying TCM

1. Discussion of Internal Factors

Internal factors, which stress vital qi, usually play the main role in any disease.

Vital qi serves as the foundation for the onset and development of disease, while pathogens are only contributing factors. The body can avoid the onset of a disease or abate its course in spite of harmful pathogens when vital qi is sufficient, while pathogens can invade the body and cause a disease or exacerbate its course when vital qi is deficient. Obviously, vital qi plays the decisive role in not just the occurrence, but also the development of a disease, while pathogens usually assume a subordinate status.

2. Holistic Medicine

This concept, viewing the various parts of the body as an organic whole, emphasizes that the interior and exterior of the body, the upper and lower parts of the body, and the left and right sides of the body are connected systematically through the channels and network vessels. This connection can be imagined as a three-dimensional network. These three dimensions include the physical, pathological, and therapeutic aspects. For example, an internally healthy body may show an exterior physiological appearance characterized by evidence such as a healthy complexion, good energetic level, stable emotions, and balanced physical movements. This indicates a healthy physiological connection. A disease that occurs in the internal organs can be seen in the exterior, through changes in color and quality of the face, tongue, pulse, and skin that indicate a pathological connection. Traditional Chinese medical treatments such as needling, massage, cupping, moxa, and ear seeding, though usually done on the exterior of the body, always heal a disorder that occurs in an internal organ. This indicates a therapeutic connection.

3. Unity of the Human Body and the External Environment

Since human beings live in an external environment, and the environment closely affects their life activities, it is apparent that a stable external environment is a basic condition for the health of human beings.

In general, the body's self-regulation mechanism allows it to acclimate to the changes that often happen in the external environment, and therefore maintain a dynamic balance between yin and yang to avoid the attack of pathogens. If the body fails to adapt to the changes in the environment, a disorder occurs.

IV. MAIN CONCEPTS OF TCM DIAGNOSTICS

Briefly, TCM diagnosis includes the four diagnostic methods of inspection, auscultation and olfaction, interrogation, and palpation and pulse examination.

The Chinese character *wàng* means "inspection" and refers to diagnosis by visual examination. This covers both general and systematic inspections. TCM puts a great deal of emphasis on inspection. The practitioner can understand not only the basic cause, but also the location, properties, and prognosis of a disorder by observing the patient's vitality[1] *(shén)*, complexion *(sè)*, physical appearance *(xíng)*, and movements and abnormalities *(tài)* in local areas of the body, including various excretory products such as sweat, sputum, saliva, urine, and stools.

The Chinese character *wén* refers to both auscultation and olfaction. Auscultation means listening to the sound and pitch of the voice, coughing, breathing, vomiting, hiccoughing, borborygmus, and groaning and speech patterns of the patient. Olfaction refers to smelling of abnormal odors emitted from either the patient or his residence. Through auscultation and olfaction, the practitioner can identify a general pattern type.

The Chinese character *wèn* means "interrogation" and refers to asking questions about how the disorder arose, its development and treatment process, what the patient feels now, the patient's and family's medical histories, individual cravings such as dietary indulgences and smoking, and the living and working conditions of the patient. The aim of interrogation is to find out the cause of the disorder and identify the pattern type by systematically uncovering the whole process of generation and development of the problem, as well as the symptoms of the patient.

The Chinese character *qiē* includes palpation and pulse examination. Palpation is the diagnostic method of palpating or pressing a certain area of the body with the practitioner's hands to find moisture and temperature changes of the skin, the shapes and characteristics of lumps, tenderness, the degree and characteristics of pain, soreness, distension, and other sensations. The frequency and rhythm of the respiration and heartbeat and the patient's reaction to palpation are also included in this category. This assists the practitioner in obtaining a general understanding of the pattern type. Pulse examination is an important method and is considered a brilliant component of TCM diagnostics. The practitioner may identify a pattern type by reading eight different qualities of each pulse including the location, frequency, length, width, strength, fluidity, tension, and equilibrium.

---

[1] Though translated elsewhere as "spirit," this can be misleading in context. In clinical application it simply refers to "life force."

V. THE PRINCIPLES OF TCM DIAGNOSIS

1. UNITY OF THE INTERIOR AND THE EXTERIOR

This approach includes two levels.

The first level is based on the holistic view of TCM that states there is unity between the interior and the exterior of the body. The body is an organic integral whole. The system of channels and network vessels links the interior and exterior of the body in both healthy and pathological states. Therefore, local physiological activities, as well as pathogenic changes, can affect the whole body; conversely, general physiologic activities and pathogenic changes can be localized in a certain area of the body. Furthermore, changes in the internal organs, qi, or blood that happen in the interior of the body can be displayed in the exterior by the condition of vitality, complexion, tongue, and pulse conditions.

The second level is based on the holistic view of TCM that states there is unity between the internal environment of the body and the external environment of nature. This means that a human body and the natural environment work together as a whole. In its normal state, the body can adapt to changes in the natural environment. A disease may occur if the regulating function of the body goes awry, or if there is an unusual change in natural conditions.

2. PATTERN IDENTIFICATION AND THE CAUSE OF DISEASE

Pattern identification is considered the essence of TCM diagnostics. Its purpose is to classify and analyze the clinical manifestations based on the four diagnostic methods and trace the causes of a disease.

The causes of disease are complex. In TCM theory, they are divided into three primary categories:

External pathogenic factors: The six environmental phenomena include wind, cold, summerheat, dampness, dryness and fire, and epidemic pathogens.

Internal pathogenic factors: The seven emotions include grief, joy, anger, anxiety/melancholy, and fear/fright.

Pathogenic factors which are neither external nor internal: These include improper food intake, fatigue, traumatic injury, sexual indulgence, and insect and animal bites.

In addition, special pathogenic factors include blood stasis, damp, phlegm, phlegm fluids, and water qi. They are produced in the course of a disease due to the dysfunction of the internal organs, and they result in additional diseases.

The clinical manifestations of a disease are dependent on the pathogenic factors involved. In the TCM view, pattern identification is the result of a comprehensive analysis of etiology, pathogenesis, and signs and symptoms of a disease in certain stages. Thus pattern identification is the main diagnostic principle and method of TCM.

3. COMPREHENSIVE APPLICATION OF THE FOUR DIAGNOSTIC METHODS

A fundamental principle of the four diagnostic methods is that they are to be used in combination. There are several reasons for this:

1) *Each diagnostic method has its limitations.* The four diagnostic methods investigate a disease from four different approaches by using several different senses including looking, listening and smelling, hearing, and touching. Each sense the practitioner uses to examine the patient is just one component. Each one has its limitations, but can focus on a specific aspect of the disease. Clinically, any one approach cannot cover all manifestations of the disease. One cannot take the place of any other. Any clinical information collected by a single method is one-sided and insufficient to correctly reflect the disease

2) *Diseases are complex.* For instance, the same disease can present different manifestations if its pattern types are different. The same manifestation can indicate different diseases if their pattern types are different. A wide-ranging examination of various aspects provides evidence for pattern identification.

3) *Manifestations are pluralistic.* For instance, the same symptom or sign such as fever, red tongue, or rapid pulse may occur in different diseases or their pattern types. Differentiating and correctly judging a disease and its pattern type is best achieved by examining a variety of aspects.

PART ONE

Diagnostic Methods

CHAPTER TWO

Inspection

Inspection refers to the diagnostic method by which the doctor observes general or local pathological changes in a patient by visual examination. Vitality, complexion, body physique and dynamic posture, tongue condition, the superficial vein of the index finger, and excretions and secretions are considered in this chapter. Inspection includes both general and systematic inspection.

I. GENERAL INSPECTION

A general inspection covers the vitality, complexion, body type, and posture and movements of the body. A general impression about the properties and severity of a disease may be obtained through general inspection.

1. VITALITY (SHÉN)

Vitality in a broad sense means the outward appearance of life activities, while in a narrow sense it refers to the spirit as such. Essence and qi of the internal organs supply vitality, so it is an external expression of the functions of the organs, essence, and qi.

The eyes, general expression, complexion, and physical characteristics of the body are the main areas of vitality inspection, among which the eyes are particularly important. The *Nei Jing (Classic of Internal Medicine)* says, "All essence and qi of the five zang organs and six fu organs flow up into the eyes."

Vitality is clinically divided into three types: Presence of vitality, absence of vitality, and false vitality, which can be compared as follows:

Presence of Vitality

Presence of vitality here refers to the general state of the essence and qi of the internal organs that is preserved without serious impairment, even while the patient is suffering from a disorder.

Absence of Vitality

Absence of vitality means that the essence and qi of the internal organs have been impaired during the course of an illness.

A comparison of signs demonstrating presence of vitality or absence of vitality is shown below in Table 2.1.

Table 2.1 Comparison between Presence and Absence of Vitality

Area of analysis	Presence of Vitality	Absence of Vitality
Eyes	Sparkle	Dull looking
Spirit	Vigorous	Listless
Facial Expression	Natural	Indifferent
Complexion	Bright, moist	Dim, dry
Mind	Clear	Confused
Speech	Correct in normal voice	Incoherent in low or high voice
Action	Coordinated	Disharmonious
Reaction	Quick	Dull
Muscle	Good muscle tone	Weak and flaccid
Severity	Mild case	Severe case
Prognosis	Good	Poor

False Vitality

False vitality usually appears in a patient whose condition is severe, or who is even dying. It manifests itself as a sudden short-lived improvement in spirit, complexion, voice, and food intake, which worsens again very soon. It indicates that the essence and qi of the internal organs are declining, leading to a separation of yin and yang. The prognosis for a patient with false vitality is usually very poor.

Presentations of false vitality are complex. The true vitality should be differentiated from a false one in clinical practice. The main presentations of false vitality are shown in Table 2.2.

Table 2.2 Presentation of False Vitality

Spirit	Complexion	Voice	Food intake
Listlessness changing to exuberance with bright eyes and a desire to meet people and to talk	Dim and dusky changing to glowing face	Low, weak and hesitant changing to loud and smooth	Lack of appetite changing to a desire to take food in larger amounts

Characteristic manifestations of false vitality are found in the appearance, duration, and stability of the patient's presentations. Characteristics of presentations of false vitality are shown in Table 2.3.

Table 2.3 Characteristics of Presentation of False Vitality

Presentation	Characteristics	Example
Appearance	Clearly seen to be unhealthy	Pale face is blushing and suffused with color as if with cosmetics
Duration	Short	Good spirits, complexion, voice, and food intake lasting a short time, then returning to the original state, or even worsening
Stability	Unstable	All false presentations are liable to change

2. COMPLEXION (SÈ)

Complexion inspection is a method of observing the color and luster of the skin to learn if there is excess or deficiency of qi and blood of the internal organs; it may also indicate the properties, severity, and prognosis of a disease.

Key Signs for Inspection

The appearance of the face.

Su Wen (Plain Questions) says: "Both qi and blood from all twelve channels and three hundred sixty-five vessels go upward to the face and cross the orifices." Therefore, the key area for complexion inspection is facial inspection. The reasons why complexion inspection is mainly limited to the face can be summed as follows:

• The blood vessels on the face are plentiful.

• The skin on the face is thinner and more tender and therefore more easily observed.

• The face is most convenient to observe.

Facial Areas Related to the Internal Organs

The facial areas related to the internal organs are the basis of complexion inspection. Thus complexion inspection takes into consideration the facial areas being observed. There are two different arrangements of facial areas. One is based on *Ling Shu (Miraculous Pivot)* (Figure 2.1), while the other is from *Su Wen (Plain Questions)* (Figure 2.2).

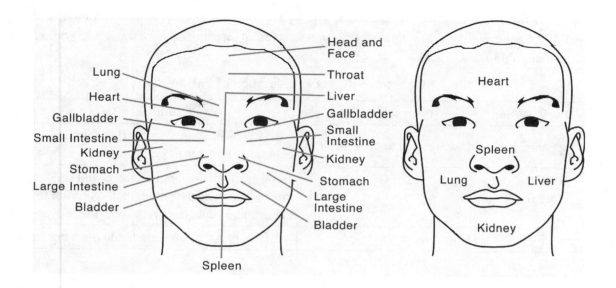

Figure 2.1 *Ling Shu* **Facial Areas Related to Internal Organs**

Figure 2.2 *Su Wen* **Facial Areas Related to Internal Organs**

Significance of Color and Luster

Complexion inspection includes observing the color and luster of the facial skin. Their clinical significances are shown in Table 2.4.

Table 2.4 Significance of Color and Luster

Items	Source	System of the Source	Physiologic Significance	Pathologic Significance
Color	Blood	Yin	Prosperity and decline of blood circulation	Property and location of a disease
Luster	Qi	Yang	Prosperity and decline of organ function	Seriousness and prognosis of a disease

Significance of Vigorous vs. Lifeless Complexion

In a pathological state, the complexion is generally divided into vigorous looking (*san se*) and lifeless looking (*wu se*). The comparison between them is shown in Table 2.5.

Table 2.5 Significance of Vigorous vs. Lifeless Complexion

Items	Manifestations	Clinical significance	Prognosis
Vigorous	Bright, moist	Mild case	Good
Lifeless	Dim, dry	Severe case	Poor

Diagnosis in Traditional Chinese Medicine

Normal Complexion

A normal complexion presents differently for different ethnic groups; for example.

• A normal complexion in Chinese and most other Asian peoples is marked by yellow suffused with red, and is moist and bright.

• A normal complexion in Caucasian people is marked by white suffused with red, and is moist and bright.

• A normal complexion includes both a main complexion *(zhǔ sè)* and a changeable complexion *(kè sè)*.

Main Complexion

The main complexion refers to the normal skin color that is consistent over the individual's lifespan.

Changeable Complexion

A changeable complexion refers to the skin color that is changeable in different external environments such as seasons, climates, place of work, place of residence, and other living conditions. Ten abnormal colorations of the complexion that can provide general information about a pattern type are listed in Table 2.6.

Table 2.6 Ten Abnormal Colorations of the Complexion

Coloration	Manifestations	Clinical Significance
Fu (Superficial)	Shallow looking	Exterior pattern
Chen (Deep)	Deep looking	Interior pattern
Qing (Clear)	Clear and smooth looking	Yang pattern
Zhuo (Pigmented)	Dusty and haggard looking	Yin pattern
Wei (Light)	Pale looking	Deficiency pattern
Shen (Dark)	Dark looking	Excess pattern
San (Dispersing)	Evenly distributed	Newly-attacking illness
Tuan (Concentrated)	Congested looking	Lingering illness process
Ze (Bright)	Bright and moist looking	Good prognosis
Yao (Dull)	Dull and dry looking	Poor prognosis

There are five abnormal colorations of the complexion that can provide more specific pathologic clues and clinical patterns, listed below in Tables 2.7–2.11.

__*White Complexion:*__ A white complexion is mainly seen in deficiency and cold patterns (see Table 2.7). Deficiency patterns include qi, blood, and yang deficiency; cold patterns include excess cold and deficiency cold, which relate to yang deficiency.

Table 2.7 White Complexion

Manifestations	Pathogenesis	Clinical Pattern
Pale white	Qi deficiency causing poor warmth and promotion of blood upward	Qi deficiency
Pale white or sallow	Blood deficiency resulting in poor nourishment of blood of the face	Blood deficiency
Suddenly turning pale	Decline of yang caused by sudden collapse of qi and blood leading to poor promotion of blood upwards	Yang exhaustion
Pale white	Bleeding leading to blood deficiency resulting in poor nourishment of the face	Qi collapse following blood collapse
Pale and puffy	Yang deficiency leading to poor warmth and promotion of blood upwards	Yang deficiency
Pale white suffused with pale blue-green	Excess cold causing contraction of the blood vessels, leading to blockage of blood circulation upwards	Excess cold

Yellow Complexion: Yellow complexion is commonly related to spleen deficiency and damp patterns (see Table 2.8).

Table 2.8 Yellow Complexion

Manifestations	Pathogenesis	Clinical Pattern
Sallow without luster	Deficiency of both qi and blood caused by hypofunction of the spleen in transportation and transformation leading to poor nourishment of the face	Spleen qi deficiency
Sallow and puffy	Spleen qi deficiency leading to production of damp retained in the body	Damp accumulation
Bright orange yellow coloration in the skin and the sclera of the eyes	Damp heat accumulating in the liver and gallbladder	Yang type jaundice
Dim yellow smoky coloration of the skin and the sclera of the eye	Cold damp disturbing the spleen and stomach	Yin type jaundice

Red Complexion: A red complexion is mainly due to a flare-up of heat regardless of whether it is excess or deficiency or false heat (see Table 2.9).

Table 2.9 Red Complexion

Manifestations	Pathogenesis	Clinical Pattern
Flushed face	Excess heat rising in the interior of the body	Excess heat
Superficial redness around zygomatic area	Deficiency heat produced by yin deficiency	Yin deficiency
Paleness intermittently suffused with blushes	Deficiency yang which is flowing outward	True cold with false heat presentation

Blue-green Complexion: A blue-green complexion is commonly related to liver wind, blood stasis, excess cold, and impediment pattern (see Table 2.10).

Table 2.10 Blue-green Complexion

Manifestations	Pathogenesis	Clinical Pattern
Blue-green or pale blue-green	Accumulation of excess cold leading to the contraction of the blood vessels, and thence to the blockage of blood circulation	Excess cold
Blue-green or gray or purple	Deficiency of heart yang leading to a blockage in the heart vessel	Impediment *(bi)*
Blue-green or purple	Blood stagnating in the vessels leading to stagnation of qi and blood	Blood stasis
Blue-green seen around the lips, on the bridge of the nose, and between the eyebrows; occurring in children	Extreme heat causing liver wind to rise	Infantile convulsion

Black Complexion: A black complexion is often found in chronic cases in which kidney deficiency, qi and blood stagnation, or phlegm and phlegm fluids accumulation may occur (see Table 2.11).

Table 2.11 Black Complexion

Manifestations	Pathogenesis	Clinical Pattern
Pale black, blue-green	Excess cold leading to contraction of blood vessels	Excess cold
Black	Stagnation of qi and blood leading to blockage of blood circulation	Impediment
Black, scaly and dry	Blood stagnating in vessels leading to poor nourishment of the skin	Blood stasis
Black and haggard	Impairment of kidney yin leading to the rise of deficiency fire and damage to yin fluids	Kidney yin deficiency
Black and puffy	Deficiency of kidney yang leading to retention of body fluids and upward rushing of turbid yin	Kidney yang deficiency
Livid rings around the eye	Yang deficiency leading to accumulation of damp and upward rushing of turbid yin (heavily descending yin damp)	Kidney yang deficiency; cold damp

3. BODY PHYSIQUE (XÍNG)

The physique of the body refers to the physical appearance of its development. In the view of TCM theory, there is no inevitable relationship between body type and diseases. But some disorders tend to occur in certain body types as shown in Table 2.12 and 2.13.

Key Signs for Inspection

Strong or weak, overweight or slender.

Table 2.12 Strong or Weak

Manifestations	Pathogenesis	Clinical significance
Strong constitution marked by thick bones, wide and thick thorax, good muscle tone, moist skin with luster	No severe impairment of qi, blood and the internal organs	Mild case with good prognosis
Weak constitution marked by thin bones, narrow and thin thorax, weak muscles and dry skin without luster	Insufficiency of qi or blood and dysfunction of the internal organs	Severe case with poor prognosis

Table 2.13 Overweight or Slender

Manifestations	Pathogenesis	Clinical Pattern
Fat, loose muscles and skin, lassitude, shortness of breath, tendency to feel tired; or easily suffering from wind stroke	Insufficiency of qi leading to its poor promotion; or damp being retained in the form of phlegm and phlegm fluids	Qi deficiency; phlegm or phlegm fluids
Emaciation, red zygomatic area, dry skin, red tongue with scant coating, thin rapid pulse, tendency of internal organs such as stomach, uterus, rectum, or even kidneys to prolapse	Impairment of yin fluids leading to production of deficiency fire	Yin deficiency

4. POSTURE AND MOVEMENTS OF THE BODY (TÀI)

The posture and movements of the body change in different illness conditions. Generally speaking, hyperactive, rapid, and excited movements usually indicate excess, heat, and yang patterns; immobility or slow and restrained movements usually indicate deficiency, cold, and yin patterns.

Key Signs for Inspection

Forced postures, loss of consciousness, and abnormal movements of the limbs and body

Forced Postures

Owing to the effects of a disorder, a patient sometimes is unable to change his position at will (see Table 2.14).

Table 2.14 Forced Postures

Manifestations	Pathogenesis	Clinical Pattern
Sitting position with the head raised, cough, asthma with sputum, rolling pulse	Phlegm accumulating in the chest leading to reversal of lung qi	Phlegm
Sitting position with the head raised, pain of the chest, fever, red tongue with yellow coating, rapid pulse	Heat accumulating in the chest leading to reversal of lung qi	Lung heat
Sitting position with the head bent, cough and asthma with weak voice	Lung qi deficiency leading to poor promotion of breathing	Lung qi deficiency

Sitting position with the head bent, cough, asthma with difficult inhalation, soreness and flaccidity of the lumbar area and knees, possible incontinence of urine	Insufficiency of kidney qi leading to inability to grasp qi	Kidney qi deficiency
Opisthotonos, high fever occurring in febrile disease	Rising of liver wind caused by extreme heat	Excess heat
Limpness, flaccidity, and atrophic muscles of the lower limbs	Insufficiency of qi and blood leading to poor nourishment of the limbs	Sequelae of cerebrovascular accident; gangrene of toe; impediment pattern and infantile paralysis

Consciousness

Consciousness may be affected in some severe and urgent cases (see Table 2.15).

Table 2.15 Consciousness

Manifestations	Pathogenesis	Clinical Pattern
Sudden loss of consciousness, cold limbs, normal respiration, no sequel after wakening	Emotional distress or extreme pain leading to upward stirring of qi and blood	Syncope
Sudden loss of consciousness, deviation of the mouth and the eyes, inability to speak, and hemiplegia after regaining consciousness	Wind phlegm obstructing the internal organs or the network vessels	Wind stroke
Sudden loss of consciousness, convulsion of the limbs, drooling with frothy saliva, wheezing, returning to normal state after regaining consciousness, as seen in epilepsy	Upward stirring of wind phlegm	Upward stirring of wind phlegm

Abnormal Movements

Inspection of different abnormal movements will help establish the diagnosis for corresponding disorders (see Table 2.16).

Diagnosis in Traditional Chinese Medicine

Table 2.16 Abnormal Movements

Manifestations	Pathogenesis	Clinical Pattern
Tremors of the eyelids, face, lips, fingers, and toes occurring in chronic illness	Insufficiency of yin and blood leading to poor nourishment of the muscles and tendons	Deficiency
Tremors of the eyelids, face, lips, fingers, and toes occurring in febrile disease	Extreme heat leading to upward stirring of liver wind	Liver wind rising
Convulsions and spasms of the limbs, rigidity of the neck and upper back, upward staring of the eyes, and possibly opisthotonos; seen in tetanus, infantile convulsions, or drug poisoning	Upward stirring of wind and toxicity	Liver wind rising

II. SYSTEMATIC INSPECTION

Systematic inspection is a diagnostic method that is based on a general inspection. By examining abnormal changes in a localized area, the general situation of an illness can be determined.

1. INSPECTION OF THE HEAD

The brain, referred to as the sea of marrow and governed by the kidney, is included in the inspection of the head. The three yang channels of the hand and foot, the du, ren and chong, as well as the liver channel of foot jue yin, all intersect on the head. The hair is the surplus of blood. Thus pathological changes occurring in the head are closely related to the state of the essence and qi of the internal organs.

Key Signs for Inspection

The shape of the head, closure of the fontanel, and appearance of the hair.

Condition of the Head

The shape and size of the head is closely related to the development of the cranial bones, so the following disorders always occur in infants (see Table 2.17).

Table 2.17 Condition of the Head

Manifestations	Pathogenesis	Clinical Pattern
Abnormally small head with incomplete development of the brain, and mental deficiency seen in congenital defects	Kidney essence deficiency leading to poor nourishment of the head	Kidney essence deficiency
Enlargement of an infant's head, mental deficiency seen in hydrocephalus	Kidney essence deficiency combined with an accumulation of phlegm fluids retained in the brain	Phlegm fluids
Caput quadratum seen in rickets	Deficiency of spleen and stomach qi leading to poor provision of qi and blood	Qi-blood deficiency
Involuntary shaking, spasm of the limbs, stiffness of the neck	Upward stirring of liver wind	Liver wind rising
Involuntary shaking, numbness of the limbs, listlessness, flaccidity of the neck	Insufficiency of qi and blood leading to poor nourishment of the head	Qi-blood deficiency

Fontanel

The fontanel refers to the space between the cranial bones. The posterior fontanel should be closed within 2-4 weeks after birth, while the anterior fontanel should be closed within 1-1.5 years and is the main area for inspection. The interpretation of an abnormal closure of the fontanel is shown in Table 2.18.

Table 2.18 Fontanel

Manifestations	Pathogenesis	Clinical Pattern
Delayed closure, five kinds of retardation and flaccidity*[2]	Kidney essence deficiency leading to poor development	Kidney essence deficiency
Delayed closure, poor appetite, sallow complexion, lassitude, weak pulse; seen in rickets	Weakness of the spleen and stomach leading to poor generation of qi and blood	Spleen qi deficiency

---

[2] The five kinds of retardation and flaccidity are the main manifestations of delayed development in infants. The former includes delayed developments in standing, walking, speech, hair growth, and teething, while the latter covers flaccidity of the neck, upper back, extremities, muscles, and mastication.

Bulging fontanel, high fever occurring in febrile diseases	Excess heat flaring upward	Excess heat
Pitting fontanel, five kinds of retardation and flaccidity	Kidney essence deficiency leading to poor development	Kidney essence deficiency
Pitting fontanel, combined with poor appetite, lassitude, listlessness, sallow complexion, abdominal distension, loose stools occurring in infantile malnutrition	Weakness of the spleen and stomach leading to poor generation of qi and blood	Spleen qi deficiency
Pitting fontanel following severe diarrhea and vomiting	Severe impairment of body fluids	Collapse of qi and yin

Hair

The growth of hair is closely related to the state of kidney qi, essence, and blood. Primary attention should be paid to the color, luster, thickness, and loss of hair and an abnormal feeling of the scalp (see Table 2.19).

Table 2.19 Hair

Manifestations	Pathogenesis	Clinical Pattern
Loss of hair, dry hair without luster occurring in chronic or consumptive cases	Insufficiency of kidney essence and blood leading to poor nourishment of the hair	Deficiency
Loss of hair occurring in young and middle-aged people, dizziness, forgetfulness, soreness and flaccidity of the lumbar area and knees	Insufficiency of kidney essence leading to poor nourishment of the hair	Kidney deficiency
Loss of hair, itching, dandruff, irritability, red tongue, rapid pulse	Flaring up of blood heat producing dryness	Blood heat
Sudden loss of hair, alopecia areata, headache, pale face and lips, floating pulse	Insufficiency of blood accompanied by attack of external wind	Blood deficiency combined with attack of external wind
Premature graying of the hair after emotional distress and overstrain, listlessness, forgetfulness, insomnia, numbness of the body, thin pulse	Insufficiency of heart blood leading to poor nourishment of the hair	Blood deficiency

Premature graying of the hair, soreness and flaccidity of the lumbar area and knees, listlessness, dizziness, and tinnitus	Insufficiency of kidney essence leading to poor nourishment of the hair	Kidney deficiency
Tangled sparse dry hair, poor appetite, loose stools, abdominal distension	Weakness of spleen and stomach leading to poor generation of qi and blood	Infantile malnutrition

2. INSPECTION OF THE FACE

In the view of TCM, essence and qi from the internal organs rise up to the face. Inspecting the face not only aids in determining the absence or presence of vitality, but also helps to identify those disorders that are related to weakness or excess of essence and qi of the internal organs.

Key Signs for Inspection

Edema, swelling, and unusual appearance.

Facial Edema

Edema occurring in the face is usually part of general edema. Facial edema is clinically divided into two types, as shown in Table 2.20.

Table 2.20 Facial Edema

Manifestations	Pathogenesis	Clinical Pattern
Edema occurring suddenly, starting with the eyelids, then spreading to the trunk and the limbs, particularly in the upper body	Wind water attacking the lung leading to failure of the lung to drain the water passages	Wind water attacking the lung (yang type edema)
Edema occurring slowly, starting with the lower limbs, then spreading to the trunk; more severe in the lower body	Deficiency of spleen and kidney yang leading to failure of the spleen and kidney to distribute and drain body fluids	Spleen-kidney yang deficiency (yin type edema)

Swelling

Facial swelling is often found with various skin infections and mumps (see Table 2.21).

Diagnosis in Traditional Chinese Medicine

Table 2.21 Facial Swelling

Manifestations	Pathogenesis	Clinical Pattern
Swollen face with painful, bright red skin in a localized area; color doesn't fade with pressure	Flaring up of wind heat or toxic fire	Erysipelas identified as excess fire/heat
Swelling around the ear lobe, pain of the parotid glands lasting a day or two, low-grade fever; seen in mumps	Upward flaring of toxic heat	Wind warm disease

Deviation of the Eyes and Mouth

Deviation of the eyes and mouth refers to a special appearance that is marked by flaccidity of the facial muscles on the affected side, the disappearance of normal forehead folds and nasolabial sulcus, inability to close the eyes, and ptosis of the labial angle. Deviation of the eyes and mouth is commonly found in facial paralysis and wind stroke pattern (see Table 2.22).

Table 2.22 Deviation of the Eyes and Mouth

Manifestations	Pathogenesis	Clinical Pattern
Sudden deviation of the eyes and mouth, inability to close the eyes, no hemiplegia; seen in Bell's palsy	Wind cold attacking upward and accumulating in the network vessels	Exterior cold
Deviation of the eyes and mouth, inability to speak, hemiplegia	Wind phlegm stirring upward and obstructing the network vessels	Wind stroke

3. INSPECTION OF THE EYES

The eyes are the opening of the liver and serve as the external indicators of the heart. Qi from the five *zang* and six *fu* organs all rises up to the eyes.

Key Signs for Inspection
Color, condition, and movements.

Five Wheel Theory

The five wheel theory states that different parts of the eye are physiologically and pathologically related to specific zang organs and the phase which represents that zang organ (see Fig. 2.3). Therefore, all eye disorders are caused by a dysfunction of the relevant zang organs. The five wheels and their related zang organs are shown in Table 2.23.

Figure 2.3 The Five Wheels and Their Related Areas

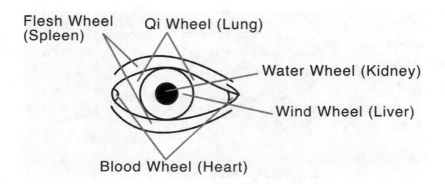

Table 2.23 The Five Wheels and Their Related Zang Organs

Wheel	Eye area	Zang organ
Flesh	Eyelid	Spleen
Qi	Bulbar conjunctiva and sclera	Lung
Blood	Inner and outer canthus	Heart
Wind	Cornea, anterior chamber, and iris	Liver
Water	Pupil and lens	Kidney

Disorders of the Five Wheels

Eyelid (Flesh Wheel)

Disorders of the eyelids are related to the spleen (see Table 2.24).

Table 2.24 Eyelid Disorders Related to the Spleen (Flesh)

Manifestations	Pathogenesis	Clinical Pattern
Redness and ulceration of the palpebral margin, occurring in blepharitis and marginalis	Damp heat accumulating in the spleen channel	Damp heat
Poor closure of the eyelids during deep sleep, occurring in chronic infantile convulsions	Spleen qi deficiency leading to poor lifting of lucid yang	Spleen qi deficiency

Diagnosis in Traditional Chinese Medicine

Prolapse of the eyelids from birth	Deficiency of both spleen and kidney qi leading to poor promotion.	Spleen qi-kidney qi deficiency
Prolapse of the eyelids, muscular atrophy and flaccidity of the limbs, occurring in myasthenia gravis	Spleen qi deficiency failing to lift lucid yang (lightly ascending yang qi)	Spleen qi deficiency
Sudden inability to close one eyelid, deviation of the eyes and mouth; occurring in Bell's palsy	Wind cold attacking and accumulating in the network vessels	Exterior cold
Inability to close the eyelids bilaterally, occurring in hyperthyroidism	Wind phlegm accumulating inside the body and stirring upward	Interior wind

Canthus (Blood Wheel)

Heart disorders often present at the canthi (see Table 2.25).

Table 2.25 Canthus Disorders Related to the Heart (Blood)

Manifestations	Pathogenesis	Clinical Pattern
Redness of the canthi, irritability, insomnia, red tip of the tongue; occurring in hyperemia	Flaring of excess heart fire	Heart fire rising

Bulbar Conjunctiva and Sclera (Qi Wheel)

The lung governs qi, so disorders occurring in these areas often involve the lung (see Table 2.26).

Table 2.26 Bulbar Conjunctiva and Sclera Disorders Related to the Lung (Qi)

Manifestations	Pathogenesis	Clinical Pattern
Bloodshot eyes with pain and discomfort; occurring in acute bulbar conjunctivitis	Wind heat attacking the liver channel and flaring upward to injure the blood vessels	Wind heat attacking the liver channel
Painful and bloodshot eyes with lumps like pomegranate seeds on the sclera; occurring in acute scleritis	Upward flaring of liver fire leading to stagnation of qi and blood	Upward flaring of liver fire

Severely bloodshot eyes without pain or discomfort; occurring in subconjunctival ecchymosis	Excess heat flaring in the lung channel and damaging the blood vessels	Lung heat
Bright yellow sclera and orange-like skin, fullness and distension of the hypochondrium, nausea, yellow greasy tongue coating, and wiry rapid pulse, occurring in yang-type jaundice	Damp heat accumulating in both the liver and gallbladder	Liver-gallbladder damp heat
Dim yellow coloring of the sclera and skin like smoke, poor appetite, white and greasy tongue coating, soggy and slow pulse; occurring in yin-type jaundice	Cold damp disturbing both the spleen and stomach	Spleen-stomach cold damp

Cornea, Anterior Chamber, and Iris (Wind Wheel)

The cornea, anterior chamber, and iris are pathologically related to the liver (see Table 2.27).

Table 2.27 Cornea, Anterior Chamber and Iris Disorders Related to Liver (Wind)

Manifestations	Pathogenesis	Clinical Pattern
Star-like spots scattered on the cornea appearing over a short time, painful eyes; occurring in non-supportive keratitis at the acute stage	Wind heat accumulating in liver channel leading to upward flaring of liver fire	Excess heat
Star-like spots scattered on the cornea appearing over a long period, discomfort of the eyes; occurring in non-supportive keratitis at the chronic stage	Flaring of deficiency fire produced by liver and kidney yin deficiency	Deficiency heat
Coagulated fat-like spots scattered near the front of the eyes; occurring in purulent keratitis	Upward flaring of liver fire and being stirring up of toxic heat accumulating in the eyes	Excess heat

Pupil and Lens (Water Wheel)

Disorders involving the pupil and lens are generally related to the kidney (see Table 2.28).

Table 2.28 Pupil and Lens Disorders Related to the Kidney (Water)

Manifestations	Pathogenesis	Clinical Pattern
Contracted pupils occurring in acute iritis, bloodshot and painful eyes, irritability, wiry rapid pulse	Liver fire flaring upward leading to liver wind	Liver fire flaring upward
Contracted pupils occurring in chronic iritis, discomfort of the eyes, five palm heat, night sweats, thin rapid pulse	Liver yin and kidney yin deficiency leading to poor nourishment of the eyes	Deficiency heat
Contracted pupils, loss of consciousness; occurring in drug or food poisoning	Toxicity leading to collapse of vital qi	Toxicity
Enlarged pupils, loss of consciousness; occurring in drug or food poisoning	Toxicity leading to collapse of vital qi	Toxicity
Enlarged pupils; occurring in severe cases or following a chronic or serious illness	Severe impairment of kidney essence and qi	Kidney essence-qi collapse
Enlarged pupils; occurring in glaucoma, with headaches and distension of the eyeballs	Qi stagnation leading to obstructed circulation of blood	Qi-blood stagnation
Icicle-like opacity, senile cataract marked by glistening opacity in the posterior capsule of the lens	Liver yin and kidney yin deficiency leading to upward flaring of deficiency fire	Liver-kidney yin deficiency

Abnormal Mobility

Under normal conditions the eyeballs move voluntarily and smoothly. Abnormal mobility is often indicative of a pathogenic disorder, as shown in Table 2.29.

Table 2.29 Abnormal Eye Mobility

Manifestations	Pathogenesis	Clinical Pattern
Protruding eye seen in tumor and cancer, occurring unilaterally	A lesion is occupying space in the eye	Qi stagnation and blood stasis
Protruding eyes seen in hyperthyroidism, occurring bilaterally	Wind phlegm accumulating internally and stirring upward	Wind phlegm
Upward staring; occurring in infantile convulsions	Extreme heat engendering wind and stirring upward	Liver wind

Downward deviation with the iris looking like the setting sun; occurring in hydrocephalus	Phlegm fluids retained in the head	Wind phlegm

4. INSPECTION OF THE EARS

The ears are the opening of the kidney. The hand shao yang and foot shao yang channels both connect to the ears, and the hand tai yang and foot tai yang and the foot yang ming channels also encircle the ears. In addition, all internal organs have their own corresponding points in the auricle. Therefore, the inspection of the ears can be used for disorders occurring almost anywhere in the body.

Key Signs for Inspection

Color, appearance, and excretions (see Table 2.30).

Table 2.30 Ears

Manifestations	Pathogenesis	Clinical Pattern
Yellow, thick pus with foul smell; occurring in acute otitis media suppurativa, with pain inside the ear	Liver-gallbladder damp heat steaming upwards	Excess heat
Clear thin pus without foul smell, vague pain of the ear; occurring in chronic otitis media suppurativa	Live and kidney yin deficiency leading to deficiency fire flaring upward	Deficiency heat
Dry and dark auricular skin occurring in protracted and severe cases	Kidney essence and yin deficiency leading to poor nourishment of the ear	Kidney essence–yin deficiency

5. INSPECTION OF THE NOSE

The nose is the opening of the lung, and the stomach channel of foot yang ming penetrates both sides of the nose. Pathogenic changes in the nose are commonly related to excess or deficiency of the lung, spleen, stomach, and other organs. They are also indicative of the severity and prognosis of an illness.

Key Signs for Inspection

Color, character, and discharge (see Table 2.31).

Diagnosis in Traditional Chinese Medicine

Table 2.31 Nose

Manifestations	Pathogenesis	Clinical Pattern
Runny nose, chills and mild fever, absence of sweat, floating tense pulse	Wind cold attacking the lung and accumulating in the opening of the lung	Exterior excess
Turbid nasal discharge with fever, mild chills, sore throat, yellow thin tongue coating, floating rapid pulse	Wind heat attacking the lung and accumulating in the opening of the lung	Exterior heat
Recurrent runny nose with clear thin discharge, caused by cold air or seasonal allergies	Lung qi deficiency leading to poor promotion of body resistance	Lung qi deficiency
Recurrent runny nose with yellow thick discharge; occurring in rhinorrhea and nasal sinusitis	Wind heat accumulating in the lung channel and obstructing the opening of the lung	Wind heat attacking the lung
Nasal bleeding; occurring in febrile diseases	Excess heat damaging the blood vessels	Lung heat
Recurrent nasal bleeding, ecchymosis and petechia; occurring in hematopathy	Spleen qi deficiency failing to keep blood circulating inside the vessels	Spleen qi deficiency
Flaring of nostrils, cough, asthma, and/or excessive spitting, fullness of the chest; occurring in acute pulmonary infections	Excess heat accumulation leading to reversal of lung qi	Lung heat
Flaring of nostrils, shortness of breath, oily sweat on the forehead, hurried pulse; occurring in severe cases	Decline of vital qi	Exhaustion

6. INSPECTION OF THE LIPS

The mouth is the opening of the spleen, and the hand yang ming and foot yang ming channels go around the lips. Therefore spleen, stomach, and large intestine disorders are often reflected on the mouth. When there is sufficient stomach qi and smooth circulation of qi and blood, the lips will be red and moist.

Key Signs for Inspection

Color, character, and mobility of the lips (see Tables 2.32, 2.33, 2.34).

Table 2.32 Lip Color

Manifestations	Pathogenesis	Clinical Pattern
Lips pale red; occurring in anemia, hemophilia	Blood deficiency leading to poor nourishment of the lips	Blood deficiency
Lips dark red; occurring in febrile diseases	Excess heat accumulating in the interior of the body	Excess heat
Lips pink or cherry-colored; occurring in carbon monoxide poisoning	Poisoning leading to stagnation of qi and blood	Qi-blood stagnation
Lips dark purple or blue-green; occurring in hypoxia	Stagnation of lung qi leading to poor promotion of blood flow	Blood stasis

Table 2.33 Lip Character

Manifestations	Pathogenesis	Clinical Pattern
Dry lips, thirst, irritability, dry stools, and scant dark urine; occurs after high fever and severe sweating	Dryness and heat impairing body fluids, leading to poor moistening of the lips	Excess heat
Dry lips, thirst, irritability, dry stools, and scant dark urine; occurs after chronic low-grade night sweats	Dryness and heat impairing body fluids, leading to poor moistening of the lips, combined with yin deficiency leading to poor nourishment of the lips	Deficiency heat
Herpes, redness, painful erosion; ulceration and swelling of lips	Damp heat accumulating in the spleen and stomach	Damp heat

Table 2.34 Lip Mobility

Manifestations	Pathogenesis	Clinical Pattern
Inability to close the mouth completely, closed eyes, loose fists, incontinence of urine and stools; indicative of wind stroke (open type) or severe cases	Decline of vital qi	Exhaustion
Closure of mouth with inability to open, closed eyes, clenched fists and teeth; occurring in wind stroke (closed type), infantile convulsions, or tetanus	Wind phlegm stirring upward and affecting in the mind	Upward stirring of wind phlegm
Deviated mouth, occurring in stroke	Wind phlegm accumulating in the network vessels	Wind phlegm

Deviated mouth occurring in Bell's palsy	Wind cold attacking the network vessels	Exterior cold
Drooling with yellow sticky saliva, bad breath, poor appetite, yellow greasy tongue coating, rolling pulse	Damp heat accumulating in the spleen and stomach	Damp heat
Repeatedly and involuntarily extending the tongue and licking the lips; occurring in high fever in children	Extreme heat causing stirring of liver wind	Liver wind

7. INSPECTION OF THE TEETH AND GUMS

The teeth are the external manifestation of the bones, which are governed by the kidney. Further, the stomach channel of foot yang ming encircles the gums. Thus inspecting the teeth and gums can provide information on kidney and stomach disorders and the state of the body fluids.

Key Signs for Inspection

External appearance, color, and luster (see Tables 2.35, 2.36).

Table 2.35 Teeth

Manifestations	Pathogenesis	Clinical Pattern
Teeth bright and dry like cobblestones, with thirst, irritability, hyperactive appetite, dry stools	Excess stomach heat leading to impairment of yin fluids	Stomach heat
Teeth dry and pale like a skeleton; occurring in chronic and severe cases	Severe impairment of kidney yin leading to poor nourishment of the teeth	Exhaustion
Loss of teeth, atrophy of the gums, discomfort of upper abdomen, red tongue with scant coating	Insufficiency of kidney yin leading to poor nourishment of the gums	Kidney yin deficiency
Loss of teeth, soreness and flaccidity of the lumbar area and knees, senility and weakness	Insufficiency of kidney essence leading to poor nourishment of the teeth	Kidney essence deficiency
Teeth clenched, fists clenched, spasms of the limbs	Wind phlegm accumulating in the network vessels, or extreme heat inducing liver wind	Liver wind

Table 2.36 Gums

Manifestations	Pathogenesis	Clinical Pattern
Pale gums, pale face, listlessness, dizziness, pale tongue, and thin pulse	Insufficiency of blood leading to poor nourishment of the gums	Blood deficiency
Redness, swelling, and pain, possibly bleeding from the gums, hyperactive appetite, bad breath	Stomach fire flaring upward and injuring blood vessels	Stomach fire
Redness, swelling, severe pain, ulceration; occurring in epidemic diseases	Toxic heat stirring upward and accumulating in the stomach channel	Toxic heat
Pale gums, atrophy of the gums	Insufficiency of stomach yin leading to poor nourishment of the gums	Stomach yin deficiency
Recurrent bleeding from the gums, ecchymosis and petechia of the limbs; occurring in hematopathy	Insufficiency of spleen qi causing failure to keep blood circulating inside the blood vessels	Spleen qi deficiency
Light red gums, slight swelling, no pain, five-palm heat, red tongue with scant coating	Insufficiency of kidney yin causing deficiency fire to flare upward and injure the blood vessels	Kidney yin deficiency

8. INSPECTION OF THE THROAT

The throat serves as a passageway for respiration and food intake, so it is related to the lung and stomach. Additionally, the kidney channel of foot shao yin goes upward to the throat and the tongue. Thus inspecting the throat can help to identify disorders of the lung, stomach, and kidney.

Table 2.37 Throat

Manifestations	Pathogenesis	Clinical Pattern
Throat dark red with severe swelling and pain; occurring in acute laryngopharyngitis	Extreme heat from the lung and stomach accumulating in the throat	Excess heat
Redness and tenderness of the throat, with slight swelling and pain	Insufficiency of lung and kidney yin producing deficiency fire flaring upward	Yin deficiency

Redness, swelling, severe pain, fever; occurring in acute tonsillitis	Excess heat from the lung and stomach accumulating in the throat	Excess heat
Soft crust (pseudo-membrane) that forms over the affected mucous membrane; when it is easy to strip off it indicates purulent tonsillitis; when it is not easy to strip off it indicates diphtheria	Toxic heat flaring upward and accumulating in the throat	Toxic heat

9. INSPECTION OF THE NECK

The large intestine channel of hand yang ming and the stomach channel of foot yang ming go through the front of the neck. The bladder channel of foot tai yang and the du channel go through the back of the neck, and the gallbladder channel of foot shao yang goes through both sides of the neck. Therefore, disorders of the organs, qi, and blood are manifested in the neck.

Key Signs for Inspection

External appearance and mobility (see Tables 2.38, 2.39).

Table 2.38 External Appearance of the Neck

Manifestations	Pathogenesis	Clinical Pattern
Enlarged and soft thyroid gland with normal skin color; occurring in goiter	Stagnated qi accumulating in the neck	Qi stagnation
One or several lumps located in the thyroid gland which can be moved by pressing; occurring in thyroid adenoma	Qi stagnation combined with phlegm accumulation	Qi stagnation-phlegm accumulation
Enlarged and hardened thyroid gland with either concave or convex surface; occurring in thyroid cancer	Qi stagnation combined with blood stasis	Qi-blood stagnation

Table 2.39 Mobility of the Neck

Manifestations	Pathogenesis	Clinical Pattern
Stiffness of the neck with limited range of motion, fever, chills, no sweating, thin white tongue coating, floating pulse	Wind cold attacking the tai yang channel leading to obstruction of qi and blood	Exterior cold
Stiffness of the neck, high fever, loss of consciousness, spasms of the limbs	Excess fire flaring upward to induce liver wind	Liver wind

Flaccidity of the neck, inability to raise the head; occurring in infants with the five kinds of retardation and flaccidity	Insufficiency of kidney essence leading to poor development	Kidney essence deficiency
Flaccidity of the neck, inability to raise the head; occurring in chronic or severe cases	Collapse of essence and qi of the internal organs	Exhaustion
Distension of the jugular vein, carotid pulsation, dizziness, headache, soreness and flaccidity of the lower back and knees; occurring in hypertension	Insufficiency of liver and kidney yin leading to rising of liver yang	Liver yang rising
Distension of the jugular vein, dark face and purple lips, stabbing pain and fullness in the chest possibly radiating to the forearm	Stagnation of heart blood or lung qi	Qi stagnation and blood stasis
Distension of the jugular vein which is aggravated in horizontal position; possibly carotid pulsation, palpitations, edema	Upsurge of kidney water causing disturbance of heart qi	Water qi intimidating the heart

10. INSPECTION OF THE CHEST

The thoracic cavity contains the heart and lung and belongs to the upper burner. The breasts are related to the stomach channel and the nipples to the liver channel. Therefore, abnormal states in the chest can reflect pathological changes of the lung, heart, liver, and stomach.

Key Signs for Inspection

External appearance, respiration (see Table 2.40).

Table 2.40 External Appearance of the Chest

Manifestations	Pathogenesis	Clinical Pattern
Flat chest, more common in slender body types	Insufficiency of both qi and yin leading to poor nourishment of the chest	Qi-yin deficiency
Barrel-shaped chest, with chronic cough, asthma with sputum; occurring in emphysema	Impairment of lung and kidney leading to lung qi accumulating in the chest	Lung-kidney deficiency

Pigeon breast, with five kinds of retardation and flaccidity	Insufficiency of kidney essence leading to poor development	Kidney essence deficiency
Pigeon breast, with lassitude, poor appetite, malnutrition	Weakness of the spleen and stomach leading to poor generation of qi and blood	Spleen-stomach deficiency
Emaciation with delayed development	Insufficiency of kidney essence and qi leading to poor development	Kidney essence-qi deficiency
Redness, swelling, sensation of heat and pain in the breast in women, possibly with ulcers, fever, and chills	Stagnated liver qi producing internal heat combined with an attack of wind heat	Excess heat
Breast tumors	Stagnation of liver qi leading to obstruction of blood circulation	Qi stagnation and blood stasis

Table 2.41 Respirations

Manifestations	Pathogenesis	Clinical Pattern
Increased thoracic breathing with decreased abdominal breathing; occurring in ascites, tumor, or pregnancy	Ascitic fluids, tumor, or fetus causing qi and blood stagnation	Indicative of abdominal disorders
Increased abdominal breathing with decreased thoracic breathing; occurring in tuberculosis, pleurisy, or thoracic trauma	Thoracic fluids, tuberculosis, and trauma causing qi and blood stagnation	Indicative of thoracic disorders
Asymmetrical breath on both sides of the chest; occurring in pleurisy and tumor	Thoracic fluids and tumor causing qi and blood stagnation	Indicative of thoracic disorders
Prolonged and difficult inhalation, rapid breathing; occurring in acute laryngopharyngitis, diphtheria	Toxic heat accumulating in the throat	Toxic heat
Prolonged and difficult exhalation; occurring in asthma, pulmonary emphysema	Insufficiency of kidney qi causing failure to grasp lung qi	Lung-kidney qi deficiency
Irregular breathing seen in chronic or severe cases	Collapse of lung qi which fails to support breathing	Qi exhaustion

11. INSPECTION OF THE ABDOMEN

The abdomen refers to the area from below the xiphoid process to above the pubis. It contains both the middle burner and lower burner and is the location of the liver, gallbladder, spleen, stomach, intestines, kidney, bladder, and uterus.

Key Signs for Inspection

Distension, concavity and subcutaneous varicose veins of the abdominal wall (see Table 2.42).

Table 2.42 Abdomen

Clinical Manifestations	Pathogenesis	Clinical Pattern
Abdominal distension, possibly emaciated limbs, fullness, hardness, subcutaneous varicose vein of abdominal wall; occurring in ascites	Stagnation of liver qi leading to blood stasis and possibly damp retention	Qi stagnation and blood stasis
Abdominal distension, general edema	Dysfunction of the lung, spleen, and kidney leading to body fluids overflowing into the muscles and skin	Fluid retention
Concave abdomen, emaciation, poor appetite, weak pulse; seen in chronic cases	Weakness of the spleen and stomach leading to poor generation of qi and blood	Spleen-stomach qi deficiency
Concave abdomen, scaly abdominal skin, muscular atrophy and flaccidity; seen in severe and chronic cases	Decline of essence and qi of the internal organs	Qi-yin exhaustion
Concave abdomen following severe vomiting and diarrhea	Impairment of body fluids	Yin exhaustion

12. INSPECTION OF THE LUMBAR AREA AND BACK

The kidney is located in the lumbar area on both sides of the spine. The *du* and bladder channels pass through the back and the *dai* channel across the lumbar area. Therefore, the inspection of the lumbar area and the back is significant in identifying disorders related to the internal organs and channels.

Key Signs for Inspection

External appearance, lateral curvature and range of motion (see Table 2.43).

Table 2.43 Lumbar Area and Back

Manifestations	Pathogenesis	Clinical Pattern
Kyphosis occurring in infants, with the five kinds of retardation and flaccidity	Insufficiency of kidney essence leading to poor development	Kidney essence deficiency
Kyphosis occurring in old age; weakness, soreness, and flaccidity of the lumbar area and knees	Insufficiency of kidney qi leading to poor promotion and nourishment of the spine	Kidney qi deficiency
Severe emaciation with vertebrae obviously exposed, occurring in chronic and severe cases	Decline of essence and qi of the internal organs	Exhaustion
Opisthotonos, stiffness of the neck, spasms of the limbs, and clenched teeth and fists	Stirring of liver wind leading to convulsions of the tendons and muscles	Liver wind
Muscular constriction of the lumbar area, pain with limited range of motion	Cold damp attacking the lower back leading to obstruction of qi and blood	Cold-damp impediment
Muscular constriction of the lumbar area, pain with limited range of motion, following traumatic injury	Trauma impairing blood vessels leading to blood stagnation in affected area	Blood stasis

13. INSPECTION OF THE LIMBS

The limbs include all four extremities and their joints and appendages, such as the fingers and toes. In zang fu theory, the heart governs blood circulation and the blood vessels, the liver governs the tendons, the kidney the bones, and the spleen the muscles and limbs. In terms of channel theory, all the hand yang and hand yin channels go through the upper limbs, and all the foot yang and foot yin channels go through the lower limbs. Therefore, disorders related to the internal organs and channels can be reflected in the limbs.

Key Signs for Inspection

External appearance and mobility of the limbs (see Table 2.44).

Table 2.44 Limbs

Manifestations	Pathogenesis	Clinical Pattern
Swollen and painful joints with limited range of motion, marked by severe pain relieved by warmth	Excess cold accumulating in the joints leading to stagnation of qi and blood	Cold impediment

Swollen and painful joints with limited range of motion, marked by local redness and hot sensation	Excess heat accumulating in the joints leading to stagnation of qi and blood	Heat impediment
Swollen and painful joints with limited range of motion, marked by heaviness of the limbs	Damp disturbing the joints leading to stagnation of qi and blood	Damp impediment
Swollen and painful joints with limited range of motion, marked by migrating pain	Wind accumulating in the joints leading to stagnation of qi and blood	Wind impediment
Knee swollen like a crane's knee with atrophy and flaccidity of the muscles	Wind damp obstructing the channels and network vessels over a long period, leading to poor nourishment of the limbs	Wind damp impediment
Flaccidity of the limbs, possibly muscular atrophy, inability to walk but absence of pain	Insufficiency of qi and blood leading to poor nourishment of the muscles and tendons	Flaccidity
Valgus or varus of the knees with the five kinds of retardation and flaccidity	Congenital defect from kidney essence deficiency	Kidney essence deficiency
Valgus or varus of the knees with pale face, poor appetite, emaciation, listlessness, and weak pulse	Acquired malnutrition caused by weakness of the spleen and stomach leading to poor generation of qi and blood	Spleen-stomach deficiency

14. INSPECTION OF THE SKIN

The skin is linked to the lung in an exterior-interior relationship, and wei qi travels through it to protect the body. The internal organs, qi, and blood also promote and nourish the skin through the channel system.

Key Signs for Inspection

Color and luster, moisture and swelling, and skin lesions (see Tables 2.45 to 2.48).

Table 2.45 Color and Luster of the Skin

Manifestations	Pathogenesis	Clinical Pattern
Redness of skin, swelling, hot sensation, and pain with sudden onset, occurring particularly in the upper body.	Wind heat attacking the skin and producing upward flaring of fire	Exterior heat

Redness of skin, swelling, hot sensation and pain, occurring particularly in the lower body.	Excess heat accumulating in the body producing upward flaring of fire	Excess heat
Skin bright yellow like an orange, accompanied by yellow sclera and urine	Damp heat accumulating in the liver and gallbladder leading to bile penetrating into the skin	Yang-type jaundice
Dim yellow smoke-like skin, accompanied by yellow sclera and urine	Cold damp accumulating in the spleen and stomach leading to bile penetrating into the skin	Yin-type jaundice
Dusky skin, particularly on the face and forehead, with soreness and flaccidity of the lumbar area and knees	Excessive strain or indulgence in sexual activity, excessive, leading to kidney yang and yin deficiency, or consumption from a chronic illness leading to kidney yang and yin deficiency	Kidney deficiency

Table 2.46 Moisture and Swelling of the Skin

Manifestations	Pathogenesis	Clinical Pattern
Scaly and dry skin	Blood stasis accompanied by blood deficiency leading to poor nourishment of the skin	Blood stasis and blood deficiency
Edema starting from the eyelids, then spreading to the trunk and limbs, particularly in the upper body	Wind water attacking the lung and penetrating into the skin and interstices of the muscles	Yang-type edema
Edema starting from the low limbs, then spreading to the trunk and face, particularly in the lower body	Insufficiency of spleen and kidney yang leading to poor transportation of water damp, then penetrating into the skin and interstices of the muscles	Yin-type edema
Dry skin seen after severe vomiting, serious diarrhea, or profuse sweating	Severe impairment of body fluids	Yin deficiency
Minute sweat blisters like millet seeds, occurring in febrile diseases	Externally attacking damp heat accumulating on the surface of the body and leading to sweat retained in the skin	Damp warm

Table 2.47 Macula and Papula

Skin Lesion	Yang Type	Yin Type
Color	Bright red	Pale red
Region of distribution	Trunk, limbs	Chest
Size	Larger	Smaller
Accompanying symptoms	Acute onset, fever, red tongue, rapid pulse	Chronic onset, no fever, pale tongue, weak pulse
Frequency of occurrence	Frequent	Seldom
Pathogenesis	Invasion of heat at the blood level compressing blood out of blood vessels	Deficiency of spleen qi leading to failure to keep blood circulating inside the vessels

Table 2.48 Other Skin Lesions

Disorder	Manifestations	Pathogenesis	Clinical Pattern
Abscess	Skin lesion with a clearly demarcated border, pain, redness, hot to the touch, swollen, and accompanied by fever	Accumulation of toxic heat	Excess heat
Yin-type carbuncle	Deep-rooted skin lesion marked by swelling without demarcation, pain and dark color in affected area; necrosis and scaling of fingers or toes as seen in thromboangitis; may occur in late stages	Accumulation of cold damp leading to stagnation of qi and blood	Yin
Yang-type carbuncle	Redness, swelling, hot sensation and pain of the affected area	Accumulation of toxic heat in the skin	Yang
Furuncle	Deep-rooted, small round skin lesion with severe pain, usually occurring on the face or fingers	Blockage of toxic heat leading to obstruction of blood circulation	Toxic heat
Boil	Small skin lesion marked by superficial redness, hot to the touch and painful	Attack of external toxic heat or accumulation of damp heat in the skin	Excess heat

III. INSPECTION OF THE SUPERFICIAL VEINS OF THE INDEX FINGER

The superficial veins of the index finger are used solely for examining infants under two years old.

1. DIAGNOSTIC THEORY

According to TCM theory, the lung channel encircles the index finger to meet with the large intestine channel, and all vessels circulate toward the lung. Therefore, the superficial veins of the index finger reflect the prevalence and decline of qi and blood of the internal organs.

2. DIAGNOSTIC METHOD

The left index finger of the infant is held with both the index finger and thumb of the practitioner's left hand. The right thumb rubs the radial surface of the infant's index finger several times from the tip to the root of the thumb to make the superficial vein more visible.

3. NORMAL APPEARANCE OF THE SUPERFICIAL VEINS OF THE INDEX FINGER

The normal appearance of the superficial veins of the index finger is light red and indistinctly visible within the wind gate. It generally traverses it diagonally, and has a single branch and an appropriate degree of thickness.

4. THE THREE GATES AND THEIR CLINICAL SIGNIFICANCE

The creases at the metacarpophalangeal articulation and interphalangeal articulations are called "gates," the first one at the base being the wind gate, the second one the qi gate, and the third one the life gate (see Fig. 2.4).

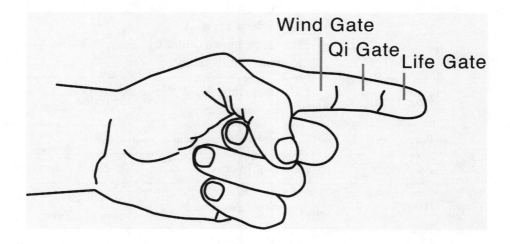

Figure 2.4 The Three Gates

The three gates theory states that the length of the superficial veins of the index finger can identify an illness. The three gates and their clinical significance are shown in Table 2.49.

Table 2.49 Three Gates and Their Clinical Significance

Length of Vein	Location of Pathogenic Factor	Clinical Pattern
Appearing between the gate of wind and the gate of qi	Exterior of the body	Exterior pattern or a mild case with a good prognosis
Extending through the gate of qi	Channels and network vessels	Interior pattern or a severe case with a poor prognosis
Crossing over the gate of life or even reaching the tip of the finger	Internal organs	Severe case with a poor prognosis

5. ABNORMAL APPEARANCE OF THE SUPERFICIAL VEINS OF THE INDEX FINGER

An abnormality of the superficial vein of the index finger may be expressed in the length, location, color, appearance, or shape of the vein (see Table 2.50).

Table 2.50 Abnormal Superficial Veins

Comparison	Manifestations	Pathogenesis	Clinical Pattern
Location	Superficial	Invasion of external pathogens	Exterior
	Deep-seated	Dysfunction of qi and blood of the internal organs or external pathogens entering the interior of the body	Interior
Color	Bright red	External pathogens attacking the exterior of the body	Exterior
	Purple-red	Stirring of internal heat	Heat
	Blue-green	Rising of liver wind	Infantile convulsions
	Black	Disturbance of blood	Severe condition with poor prognosis
Degree of coloration	Mild	Insufficiency of vital qi	Deficiency; mild case
	Strong	Exuberance of pathogens	Excess; severe case

Appearance	Increasing length	Worsening condition	Aggravating turn
	Decreasing length	improving condition	Favorable turn
	Thickening	Heat accumulating in the interior of the body	Heat or excess
	Thinning	Insufficiency of vital qi or cold congealing in the blood vessels	Cold or deficiency
Shape	Tending to slant with a single branch	Smooth circulation of blood	Mild case
	Curved or ring-like with several branches	Blockage of the blood flow	Severe case

IV. TONGUE INSPECTION

Tongue inspection is an essential part of TCM diagnostics, and is considered to be one of the most brilliant components of TCM.

1. DIAGNOSTIC THEORY

The essence and qi of all five zang and six fu organs, in particular those of the heart, stomach, and spleen, are directly or indirectly related to the tongue through the channel and collateral systems. In the view of TCM, the tongue serves as the opening of the heart and the external expression of the spleen. Moreover, stomach qi produces the tongue coating. Thus, qi and blood of the internal organs physiologically nourish the tongue while it reflects pathogenic changes in the qi and blood of the internal organs.

2. CLINICAL SIGNIFICANCE

Observation of the tongue condition may help the practitioner to learn about the location, properties, and development and prognosis of a disease. It can therefore assist in pattern identification.

3. TONGUE AREAS RELEVANT TO THE INTERNAL ORGANS

Tongue areas relevant to the internal organs are shown in Table 2.51 and Fig. 2.5.

Table 2.51 Tongue Areas

Area	Internal Organ
Tip	Heart and lung
Edges	Liver and gallbladder
Middle	Spleen and stomach
Root	Kidney

Figure 2.5 Tongue Areas Relevant to the Internal Organs

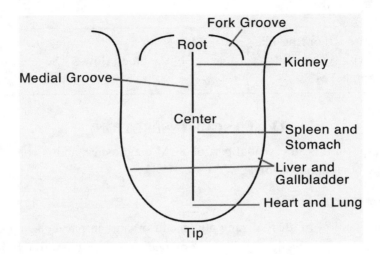

4. KEY SIGNS FOR TONGUE INSPECTION

In inspecting the tongue, the practitioner should pay particular attention to the following points:

Light

Tongue observations should be performed with natural light to avoid misinterpretation of the color.

Position and Posture of the Patient

The patient should sit comfortably with the whole body relaxed, and then stretch out the tongue with the tip downward, so that the tongue is naturally exposed.

Confusion of Tongue Coating

Some foods may discolor the tongue coating. For instance, rough foods cause the tongue coating to thin; milk may make the coating white and greasy; peanuts, seeds, beans, peach pits, or almonds and other foods which are rich in lipids may cause the coating to look greasy or curd-like. Coffee, grape juice, wine, or salty olives always stain the coating brown or dark yellow. Some drugs can also discolor the tongue coating. For instance, *wu mei (fructus mume)* or *bin lang (semen arecae catechu)* can stain the tongue coating black; *huang lian (rhizoma coptidis)* and Vitamin B$_2$ may stain it yellow; herbal decoctions may stain it yellow or brown.

Tongue Inspection Components

There are two components that must be examined in tongue inspection.

Tongue Coating

Inspection of the tongue coating is concerned with the color, thickness, moisture, root-scraping, peeling, character, and distribution of the coating on the tongue.

Tongue Body

Inspection of the tongue body is concerned with the color, quality, complexion, and movement of the tongue body, and the veins underneath the tongue.

5. Normal Tongue Condition

The normal tongue condition is light red, covered by a thin white coating that is moist. The tongue body can move voluntarily.

6. Abnormal Tongue Condition

An abnormal tongue condition may be reflected in both the tongue coating and the tongue proper.

Inspection of the Tongue Coating

In an illness, the tongue coating is generated from stomach qi that is left over from digestion. It steams upward as turbid damp and ascends to the tongue.

Key Signs for Inspection

The following categories should be observed: thickness (thin or thick), moisture content (moist or dry), character (curd-like or greasy), color and luster, root scraping, and peeling condition.

Thickness of the Tongue Coating

The thickness of the tongue coating reflects the location, advance, or retreat of a disease (see Table 2.52).

Table 2.52 Thickness of the Tongue Coating

Manifestations	Pathogenesis	Clinical Pattern
Thin	External pathogens attacking the exterior of the body	Exterior

Thick	Internal injury due to dysfunction of the internal organs	Interior
Thin coating becoming thick	Advance of the disease	Aggravated outcome
Thick coating becoming thin	Retreat of the disease	Favorable outcome

Moisture of the Tongue Coating

The moisture of the tongue coating is determined by the ascent of body fluids. It indicates whether body fluids are impaired or not (see Table 2.53).

Table 2.53 Moisture of Tongue Coating

Degree of Moisture	Pathogenesis	Clinical Pattern
Moist	No impairment of body fluids	Mild case
Watery	Disturbance by damp and retention of body fluids	Yang deficiency; damp
Dry	Impairment of body fluids	Dryness; heat; yin exhaustion

Character of the Tongue Coating

The character of the tongue coating refers to the texture, structure, and external appearance of the tongue coating. In general, there are two characters of tongue coatings. One is curd-like and is marked by a loose structure with rough particles so that the coating looks like bean dregs. The other is a greasy coating that looks like greasy fat with a compact texture and fine particles (see Table 2.54).

Table 2.54 Character of Tongue Coating

Character	Pathogenesis	Clinical Pattern
Curd-like	Accumulation of phlegm damp accompanied by excess heat, but heat is greater than damp	Phlegm heat; damp heat; stagnation of food producing heat
Greasy	Accumulation of phlegm damp accompanied by disturbed yang qi, but damp is greater than heat	Damp; phlegm; stagnation of food

Color of the Tongue Coating

Among the different aspects of an inspection of the tongue coating, color has the most clinical relevance (see Table 2.55).

Table 2.55 Color of Tongue Coating

Manifestations	Pathogenesis	Clinical Pattern
Thin, white	Invasion of wind cold	Exterior cold
Thin, watery	Accumulation of cold damp	Cold damp
Greasy, white	Disturbance by damp phlegm	Phlegm damp
Thick, greasy	Disturbance by damp or stagnation of food	Damp; food stagnation
Thin, yellow	Invasion of wind heat	Exterior heat
Thick, yellow	Accumulation of damp heat	Interior heat
Greasy, yellow	Accumulation of damp heat	Damp heat
Grey, moist	Accumulation of phlegm, phlegm fluids or cold damp	Damp; phlegm or phlegm fluids
Grey, dry	Excess or deficiency heat leading to the impairment of body fluids	Yin deficiency
Black, moist	Insufficiency of yang qi leading to the production of internal cold	Yang deficiency
Black, dry	Extreme heat leading to the exhaustion of body fluids	Yin exhaustion
Cracked	Excess interior heat leading to impairment of body fluids	Excess heat; deficiency heat

Scraping the Tongue Coating

Scraping is also referred to as root scraping. The TCM practitioner usually examines the patient by scraping the tongue coating. If some coating remains after scraping, it is said that the tongue coating is rooted (see Table 2.56).

Table 2.56 Scraping the Tongue Coating

Manifestations	Pathogenesis	Clinical Significance
Coating remains after scraping	Presence of stomach qi	Mild case with good prognosis
Coating disappears after scraping	Decline of stomach qi	Severe case with poor prognosis

Peeling of the Tongue Coating

Peeling refers to the condition whereby some or all of the tongue coating naturally disappears due to a chronic illness. The peeled area may be shaped like a chicken heart or a map, or, if all the tongue coating has peeled, it may be mirror-like (see Table 2.57).

Table 2.57 Peeling of the Tongue Coating

Manifestations	Pathogenesis	Clinical Pattern
Scattered, map-like, or chicken heart-shaped peeling, occurring in a chronic disorder	Impairment of both stomach qi and stomach yin	Qi-yin deficiency
Mirror-like peeling, occurring in severe or even critical cases	Exhaustion of stomach qi and stomach yin	Qi-yin exhaustion

Inspection of the Tongue Proper

Key Signs for Inspection

Color and luster, character, shape, texture, mobility, and veins underneath the tongue.

Table 2.58 Color and Luster of the Tongue Proper

Manifestations	Pathogenesis	Clinical Pattern
Pale	Insufficiency of qi leading to poor promotion of blood flow	Qi deficiency
	Insufficiency of blood leading to poor nourishment of the tongue	Blood deficiency
	Insufficiency of yang leading to poor warmth of blood flow	Yang deficiency
Redness on tip or edges	Heat accumulating in the heart, lung, liver, and gallbladder	Heat
Red with yellow coating	Heat accumulating inside the body	Excess heat
Red with scant or peeled coating	Yin deficiency leading to deficiency heat	Deficiency heat
Scarlet and stiff, occurring in warm disease	Extreme heat entering yin and blood levels	Toxic heat
Purple including pale purple, purple red or purple spots on the whole tongue or on the edge of the tongue	Blockage of blood circulation	Blood stasis

Table 2.59 Character of the Tongue Proper

Manifestations	Pathogenesis	Clinical Pattern
Dry and rough	Excess heat combined with impairment of body fluids	Excess heat
Tender and moist	Stagnation of yang qi inside the body	Deficiency cold
Cracked and pale	Deficiency of both qi and blood	Deficiency
Cracked and red	Impairment of body fluids due to heat	Yin deficiency
Plump, tender, and pale	Insufficiency of both spleen and kidney yang	Spleen yang-kidney yang deficiency
Plump, blue-green, and dark; occurring in drug, food, or alcohol poisoning	Toxic heat entering the heart	Toxicity
Plump, puffy, and dark	Heat accumulating in the heart and spleen	Excess heat
Pale tongue with tooth marks	Insufficiency of spleen yang leading to poor transportation of body fluids	Spleen yang deficiency
Thin and pale	Insufficiency of both qi and blood leading to poor nourishment and circulation of blood	Qi-blood deficiency
Thin and dark	Insufficient heat leading to impairment of body fluids	Deficiency heat

Table 2.60 Mobility of the Tongue Body

Character	Main Accompanying Manifestations	Pathogenesis	Clinical Pattern
Stiff tongue with dry coating	High fever, delirium, and loss of consciousness	Excess heat penetrating the pericardium and impairing body fluids	Heat
Flaccid tongue with dry and dark coating	Fever, irritability, thirst, constipation	Extreme impairment of body fluids due to heat	Heat

Stiff tongue	Deviation of the mouth and eyes; occurring in Bell's palsy	Wind cold invading the network vessels leading to stagnation of qi and blood	Exterior cold
	Deviation of the mouth and eyes, difficult speech, and hemiparalysis	Wind phlegm accumulating in the network vessels leading to stagnation of qi and blood	Wind stroke
Flaccid, moist, and pale toongue	Pale face and lips, listlessness, lassitude, weak pulse	Insufficiency of qi and blood leading to poor nourishment	Qi-blood deficiency
Tremors and stiffness	Spasms or tremors of the limbs, aching, headache, chills	External wind invading and inducing internal wind	Wind
Tremors, dryness and redness	High fever, irritability, possibly coma and delirium, thirst	Extreme heat leading to stirring up of liver wind	Liver wind
Tremors and paleness	Pale face and lips, listlessness, lassitude	Deficiency of qi, blood, and yang leading to poor nourishment and circulation of blood	Deficiency
Repeatedly and involuntarily extending the tongue and licking the lips	Fever, restlessness, spasms of the limbs; occurring in infantile convulsions	Upward stirring of spleen and heart heat	Liver wind

Table 2.61 Veins underneath the Tongue

Manifestations	Pathogenesis	Clinical Pattern
Veins appear thin, short, light red with less branching	Insufficiency of qi and blood leading to poor filling of blood vessels	Qi-blood deficiency
Veins appear thick purple or dark blue with branching; occurring in severe or even critical cases	Exhaustion of stomach qi and yin	Qi-yin exhaustion

Diagnosis in Traditional Chinese Medicine

CHAPTER THREE

Auscultation and Olfaction

This diagnostic method includes two parts: auscultation and olfaction. A patient's voice, speech, breathing, coughing, vomiting, hiccups, belching, sighing, and the unique odors of a patients' secretions and excretions all are related to the patient's physiological activities and pathological changes. The information gained from listening and smelling to detect changes in these activities can help to identify a disorder, its pattern type, and a patient's general constitutional situation.

I. AUSCULTATION

Auscultation refers to listening for abnormal sounds from the patient. Voice, speech, breathing, coughing, vomiting, hiccups, belching, and sighing will be discussed in this section in detail.

1. VOICE

The pathological changes in voice can help to identify the properties of a disease, such as cold, heat, deficiency or excess.

Key Signs for Auscultation

General state of the voice, hoarseness and loss of voice, snoring and groaning (see Tables 3.1 to 3.5).

Table 3.1 General Auscultation

Manifestations	Pathogenesis	Clinical Pattern
Loud, coarse voice	Pathogens attacking the lung leading to stagnation of lung qi	Excess
Weak, low voice	Insufficiency of lung qi leading to poor promotion of voice	Deficiency

Table 3.2 Low and Deep Voice

Manifestations	Pathogenesis	Clinical Pattern
Low and deep voice with stuffy nose, runny nose, floating pulse	External pathogens attacking the lung leading to obstruction of lung qi	Exterior excess

Table 3.3 Hoarseness and Loss of Voice

Manifestations	Pathogenesis	Clinical Pattern
Sudden hoarseness or loss of voice, fever, sore throat, rapid floating pulse	Wind heat attacking the lung and accumulating in the throat	Exterior heat
Sudden hoarseness or loss of voice, cough with sputum, fullness of the chest, malar flush	Turbid phlegm accumulating in the lung leading to poor dispersing action of the lung	Phlegm
Gradually increasing hoarseness and possibly loss of voice	Insufficiency of lung and kidney yin leading to poor nourishment of the throat	Lung yin-kidney yin deficiency

Table 3.4 Snoring

Manifestations	Pathogenesis	Clinical Pattern
Snoring occurring in chronic nasal disorders, with overweight disorders, or due to poor sleeping position	Chronic disorders of the nose, improper posture during sleep leading to interference with the passage of breath	Lung qi stagnation
Snoring with loss of consciousness, high fever, flushed face	Extreme heat penetrating the pericardium and affecting the mind	Excess heat
Frequent snoring occurring in chronic and severe cases or in loss of consciousness	Decline of vital qi leading to separation of yin and yang	Exhaustion

Table 3.5 Groaning

Manifestations	Pathogenesis	Clinical Pattern
Groaning in high and forceful voice, severe pain and distension	Attack of pathogens, stagnation of qi and blood	Excess
Groaning in low and weak voice	Insufficiency of qi, blood, yin, or yang leading to poor promotion and nourishment of sound production	Deficiency

2. Speech

Speech is one of the life activities governed by the mind, so abnormal speech is commonly related to the heart.

Key Signs for Auscultation

General state of speech and deranged speech (see Tables 3.6, 3.7).

Table 3.6 General Auscultation

Manifestations	Pathogenesis	Clinical Pattern
Desire to speak, restlessness, or deranged speech in a loud and coarse voice	Prevalence of pathogenic factors leading to excitement of the mind	Excess
No desire to speak, indifference, or deranged speech in a weak, low, and incoherent voice	Insufficiency of vital qi leading to the poor promotion of the mind	Deficiency
Speech that is weak, low, and incoherent, occurring in severe cases	Collapse of vital qi leading to poor nourishment and promotion of the mind	Exhaustion

Table 3.7 Deranged Speech

Manifestations	Pathogenesis	Clinical Pattern
Deranged speech with a sharp loud voice, restlessness, loss of consciousness	Extreme heat penetrating the pericardium or excess heat causing accumulation of dry stools in the yang ming bowels	Ying level; yang ming bowel
Deranged speech incoherently repeated in a weak and low voice, loss of consciousness	Severe impairment of heart qi leading to poor nourishment of the mind	Heart qi deficiency
Deranged speech with a sharp voice, emotional or bizarre behavior, irritability, loss of consciousness	Qi stagnation causing upstirring of phlegm fire affecting the mind	Excess heat
Deranged speech in a low voice, indifference, emotional depression, patient mutters to self, but stops speaking when meeting people; loss of consciousness; occurring in senile dementia	Insufficiency of heart qi leading to poor promotion of the mind	Heart qi deficiency

Deranged speech with a low voice, indifference and/or muttering; loss of consciousness, lassitude, heaviness of the body, greasy tongue coating; occurring in epilepsy	Stagnation and upward stirring of phlegm damp affecting the mind	Phlegm damp
Deranged speech in a low voice, indifference and/or emotional depression with frequent sighing, muttering, loss of consciousness, stabbing pain in a certain area of the body; occurring in hysteria or after cerebrovascular accidents	Stagnation of blood and qi misting the mind	Qi stagnation and/or blood stasis

3. BREATHING

Disorders manifested by abnormal respiration are mainly related to the lung.

Key Signs for Auscultation

General state of breathing, asthma, gasping breathing, shortness of breath, and weak breath (see Tables 3.8 to 3.11).

Table 3.8 General Auscultation

Manifestations	Pathogenesis	Clinical Pattern
Rapid breath with coarse, loud sounds, fullness of the chest	Excessive pathogens attacking the lung leading to stagnation of lung qi	Excess
Shortness of breath with low, weak sounds	Insufficiency of lung qi leading to poor promotion of breathing	Deficiency

Table 3.9 Asthma

Manifestations	Pathogenesis	Clinical Pattern
Asthma marked by rapid and difficult respiration with coarse sounds, possibly flaring of nostrils, open mouth, shoulders raised following inspiration, inability to lie flat, fullness of the chest, fever	Phlegm heat accumulating in the lung leading to reversal of lung qi	Lung heat

Asthma marked by rapid and difficult respiration with weak, low sounds, aggravated by exercise	Insufficiency of lung and kidney qi leading to inability to grasp qi	Qi deficiency
Asthma marked by rapid and difficult respiration with coarse sounds, wheezing	Phlegm retained in the chest accompanied by external pathogens attacking the lung	Exterior pattern combined with phlegm

Table 3.10 Gasping Breathing

Manifestations	Pathogenesis	Clinical Pattern
Gasping, coughing, asthma, frequent spitting, inability to lie down	Phlegm fluid accumulating in the chest leading reversal of lung qi	Phlegm fluids
Gasping, coughing, sore throat, five-palm heat, night sweats, red tongue with scant coating, thin rapid pulse	Insufficiency of lung yin leading to flaring of deficiency fire	Yin deficiency
Gasping, coughing, edema starting with the eyelids and face, then spreading throughout the whole body, floating pulse	External pathogens attacking the lung leading to dysfunction of the lung in dredging the water passages	Wind water attacking the lung

Table 3.11 Shortness of Breath

Manifestations	Pathogenesis	Clinical Pattern
Shortness of breath marked by shallow and rapid breathing with coarse sounds, fullness of the chest, coughing, profuse sputum	Phlegm or phlegm fluids accumulating in the chest and disturbing the flow of lung qi	Phlegm
Shortness of breath marked by shallow rapid breathing, weak sounds, listlessness, weak pulse	Insufficiency of vital qi or weak constitution	Qi deficiency
Shortness of breath with weak and low sounds but without gasping	Insufficiency of lung qi leading to poor promotion of respiration	Lung qi deficiency

4. COUGHING

Coughing is caused by reversal of lung qi. It is not only brought about by lung disorders, but is also found in disorders occurring in other internal organs, if they involve the lung.

Key Signs for Auscultation

General nature of coughing, sound, presence or lack of sputum, and accompanying manifestations (see Tables 3.12, 3.13).

Table 3.12 General Auscultation

Manifestations	Pathogenesis	Clinical Pattern
Cough with loud and explosive sounds	Excessive pathogens	Excess
Cough with weak and low sounds	Insufficiency of lung qi leading to poor promotion of sound production	Deficiency

Table 3.13 Coughing

Manifestations	Pathogenesis	Clinical Pattern
Cough with low and stuffy voice accompanied by white thin sputum and stuffy nose	Invasion of external wind cold leading to obstruction of lung qi	Exterior cold
Cough with low voice, profuse sputum, easy expectoration	Damp phlegm accumulating in the lung leading to lung qi stagnation	Damp phlegm
Cough with high and even sharp voice, profuse thick yellow sputum	Heat accumulating in the lung leading to consumption of body fluids	Excess heat
Dry cough with little or no sputum which occurs in autumn, with fevers, chills, floating pulse	Invasion of the lung by dryness	Exterior dryness
Dry cough with little or no sputum which occurs in any season, with five-palm heat, red zygomatic area, night sweats, thin rapid pulse	Insufficiency of lung yin leading to poor nourishment of voice	Deficiency heat

Whooping cough with paroxysmal loud sounds, and even bloody sputum	Attack of external wind accompanied by deep-seated phlegm	Wind phlegm heat
Cough with barking sound	Insufficiency of lung and kidney yin accompanied by toxic heat accumulating in the throat	Yin deficiency combined with toxic heat
Cough with weak voice and foamy sputum, shortness of breath, listlessness and lassitude	Insufficiency of lung qi leading to poor promotion of voice	Qi deficiency
Cough aggravated at night	Insufficiency of lung and kidney yin leading to poor nourishment of voice	Yin deficiency
Cough aggravated at dawn	Deficiency of lung and spleen yang leading to poor promotion of lung qi	Yang deficiency

5. VOMITING

Vomiting is a result of reversal of stomach qi. It can occur in any disorder that causes a failure of stomach qi to descend.

Key Signs for Auscultation

Sound; character, odor, and accompanying manifestations of the vomiting (see Tables 3.14, 3.15).

Table 3.14 General Auscultation of Vomiting

Manifestations	Pathogenesis	Clinical Pattern
Vomiting with loud, coarse sounds	Pathogens attacking the stomach leading to reversal of stomach qi	Excess
Vomiting with weak, low sounds	Insufficiency of stomach qi leading to poor promotion of voice	Deficiency

Table 3.15 Character of Vomiting

Manifestations	Pathogenesis	Clinical Pattern
Vomiting foul liquid or undigested food, abdominal pain, tenderness, thirst, bitter taste in mouth	Stagnation of food producing internal heat accumulating in the stomach	Stomach heat
Vomiting with weak sounds, spitting clear liquid, vague pain in the abdomen with preference for pressure and warmth, loose stools, and listlessness	Insufficiency of spleen and stomach yang leading to poor warmth and digestive promotion	Deficiency cold
Sudden and severe vomiting and diarrhea with white turbid liquid	Damp heat accumulating in the stomach and intestines leading to impairment of qi and blood	Damp heat
Vomiting, fullness and distension of the abdomen, constipation	Accumulation of both excessive and dry feces leading to reversal of turbid stomach qi	Excess heat
Vomiting, mental depression, hiccups, distension of the hypochondrium	Liver qi transversely attacking the stomach leading to reversal of stomach qi	Liver qi attacking the stomach

6. HICCUPS

Hiccups are from reversal of stomach qi urgently rushing outward through the throat, followed by a loud and short sound.

Key Signs for Auscultation

Sound, character, and accompanying manifestations (see Tables 3.16, 3.17).

Table 3.16 General Auscultation of Hiccups

Manifestations	Pathogenesis	Clinical Pattern
Hiccups with loud, coarse sounds	Pathogenic factors attacking the stomach and stagnating in the stomach leading to reversal of stomach qi	Excess
Hiccups with weak, low sound	Insufficiency of stomach qi leading to poor promotion of sound production	Deficiency

Table 3.17 Character of Hiccups

Manifestations	Pathogenesis	Clinical Pattern
Loud hiccups, recent onset of illness, bad breath, red tongue with yellow coating	Heat attacking the stomach leading to reversal of stomach qi	Stomach heat
Loud hiccups, abdominal pain relieved by warmth, preference for hot drinks, pale tongue with white coating	Cold attacking the stomach leading to reversal of stomach qi	Stomach cold
Frequent weak hiccups; occurring in chronic and severe cases	Collapse of stomach qi	Exhaustion

7. BELCHING

Belching is also a result of reversal of stomach qi.

Key Signs for Auscultation

Sound; character and accompanying manifestations of belching (see Tables 3.18, 3.19).

Table 3.18 General Auscultation of Belching

Manifestations	Pathogenesis	Clinical Pattern
Loud, coarse belching	Pathogenic factors attacking the stomach and stagnating, leading to reversal of stomach qi	Excess
Weak, low belching	Insufficiency of stomach qi leading to poor promotion of sound production	Deficiency

Table 3.19 Character of Belching

Manifestations	Pathogenesis	Clinical Pattern
Frequent loud belching, with sour-smelling bad breath, fullness and distension of the upper abdomen	Stagnation of undigested food leading to reversal of stomach qi	Food stagnation
Belching, usually induced by emotional depression, distension of the upper abdomen and hypochondriac region relieved after belching	Stagnated liver qi attacking the stomach leading to reversal of stomach qi	Liver qi stagnation

Frequent belching, pain in the upper abdomen, preference for warmth, expectoration of clear saliva	Cold attacking the stomach leading to reversal of stomach qi	Stomach cold
Belching with a weak voice, poor appetite; occurring in the elderly, those with weak constitution, or chronic cases	Insufficiency of spleen and stomach qi leading to poor promotion of sound production	Spleen-stomach qi deficiency

8. SIGHING

Sighing occurs to relieve discomfort of the chest and hypochondrium when emotions are depressed. It is mainly caused by stagnation of liver qi.

Key Signs for Auscultation

Frequency and accompanying manifestations (see Table 3.20).

Table 3.20 Sighing

Manifestations	Pathogenesis	Clinical Pattern
Frequent sighing usually induced by emotional depression, fullness of the upper abdomen and the hypochondrium	Stagnated liver qi stirring upward	Liver qi stagnation

II. OLFACTION

Olfaction refers to smelling the unique odors of a patient's secretions and excretions (see Table 3.21), such as breath, sweat, sputum, nasal discharge, stools, urine, menses, vaginal discharge, and vomit.

The information collected from smelling can help to identify the properties of a disorder. For instance, strong sour and foul smells usually indicate an excess heat pattern, while mild abnormal smells are always seen in a deficiency cold pattern.

Table 3.21 Abnormal Odors

Manifestations	Pathogenesis	Clinical Pattern
Foul odor from nasal passage, possibly headaches, occurring in sinusitis	Excess heat accumulating in the lung channel	Wind heat
Bad breath, toothache, gum bleeding with hyperactive appetite, occurring in gingivitis	Flaring of stomach fire	Stomach fire

Bad breath, fever, sore throat, possibly constipation, rapid pulse; occurring in tonsillitis	Toxic heat accumulating in the throat	Excess heat
Bad breath, chest pain, sputum with pus and blood; occurring in pulmonary abscess	Toxic heat accumulating in the lung	Lung heat
Vomiting undigested food with sour and foul odor; occurring in food stagnation	Stagnated food transforming into heat	Food stagnation
Foul and yellow sweat; occurring in chronic cases	Damp heat steaming outward	Spleen-stomach damp heat
Foul sweat; occurring in acute febrile diseases or warm diseases	Excess heat steaming outward	Excess heat
Foul-smelling menses of thick consistency, dark red color and clots	Downward flow of excess heat	Excess heat
Yellow and sticky leukorrhea with bad odor	Downward flow of liver and gallbladder damp heat	Damp heat
Irritating odor like rotten apples in the patient's residence; occurring in diabetes at the late stage	Outgoing of collapsed kidney qi	Kidney qi exhaustion
Acrid-smelling urine, edema; occurring in uremia at the late stage	Outgoing of collapsed kidney qi	Kidney qi exhaustion

CHAPTER FOUR

Interrogation

Symptoms are the body's reactions to pathologic changes, and serve as evidence for pattern identification. Interrogation not only means asking about the main symptoms, but also any related conditions, such as complicating symptoms. In TCM history, the famous "Ten Questions" refer to the central questions that the practitioner asks a patient to collect basic information for the diagnosis of an illness.

I. AVERSION TO COLD AND FEVER

In general, an aversion to cold can be caused by prevalence of yin or insufficiency of yang; while fever indicates a prevalence of yang or insufficiency of yin. There are four types of aversion to cold and fever in clinical practice. They are: aversion to cold accompanied by fever, aversion to cold without fever, fever without aversion to cold, and alternating attacks of fever and chills. They each indicate different patterns. We will discuss their characteristics and clinical significance one by one.

1. AVERSION TO COLD

Aversion to cold is a general concept which consists of three symptoms: chills, aversion to wind, and intolerance to cold. The comparison is shown in Table 4.1.

Table 4.1 Aversion to Cold

Manifestations	Characteristics	Clinical Pattern
Chills	Aversion to cold not relieved by warmth, often accompanied by fever. In general, fever occurs if vital qi wins, and chills occur if the pathogens win.	Exterior excess; exterior heat
Aversion to wind	Aversion to cold occurring in a windy |environment, possibly accompanied by fever	Exterior deficiency
Intolerance of cold	Aversion to cold never accompanied by fever, cold limbs, pain relieved by warmth	Excess cold; deficiency cold

2. AVERSION TO COLD ACCOMPANIED BY FEVER

Among the three types of aversion to cold, only chills accompanied by fever and chills only occur in cases of exterior pattern. It is, in fact, the characteristic symptom for diagnosing an exterior pattern. In TCM theory, it indicates that the body is resisting invasion of eternal pathogenic factors. Clinically, there are three kinds of chills accompanied by fever. They are shown in Table 4.2.

Table 4.2 Aversion to Cold Accompanied by Fever

Manifestations	Pathogenesis	Clinical Pattern
Chills greater than fever, absence of sweating, headaches, thin white tongue coating, and floating tense pulse	Invasion of external cold leading to tightness of the muscular interstices, brought about by a failure of wei qi to warm the exterior of the body	Exterior excess
Fever greater than chills, sore throat, thin yellow tongue coating, and floating rapid pulse	Invasion of external heat leading to accumulation of wei qi in the exterior of the body	Exterior heat
Chills occurring in windy environment (i.e., aversion to wind), involuntary sweating, accompanied by mild fever	External wind attacking the exterior of the body leading to looseness of the muscular interstices	Exterior deficiency

3. AVERSION TO COLD WITHOUT FEVER

An aversion to cold without fever refers to a condition in which the patient feels cold, but has a normal body temperature. It is clinically divided into two types depending on the onset and illness duration. The manifestations are shown in Table 4.3.

Table 4.3 Aversion to Cold without Fever

Manifestations	Pathogenesis	Clinical Pattern
Aversion to cold, listlessness, cold limbs, vague pain relieved by warmth and pressure, chronic illness, and deep slow weak pulse	Constitutional yang deficiency leading to poor warmth of the body surface	Deficiency cold
Aversion to cold, pain and cold sensation of abdomen or other areas, relieved by warmth but aggravated by pressure, short-term illness, and deep-slow and strong pulse	Cold invading the internal organs and damaging yang qi	Excess cold

4. FEVER WITHOUT AVERSION TO COLD

Fever means that the body temperature is higher than normal or that the body temperature may be normal but the patient feels hot either in a localized area or throughout the whole body. It can be caused either by an invasion of external pathogens or by a dysfunction of the internal organs leading to the production of internal heat.

Fever is clinically classified into high fever, tidal fever, and mild fever.

High Fever

The body temperature is over 102°F, and it is usually accompanied by malar flush, irritability, profuse sweating, and thirst with preference for cold drinks. It is caused by excess heat accumulating in the body and flowing outward.

Tidal Fever

Tidal fever refers to a fever that occurs in such a way that the temperature rises and falls regularly like the tide. In clinical practice, there are three kinds of tidal fever as shown in Table 4.4.

Table 4.4 Tidal Fever

Manifestation	Pathogenesis	Clinical Pattern
Tidal fever occurring in the afternoon or night fever with red zygomatic area, night sweats, five-palm heat, red tongue with scant coating, and thin rapid pulse	Yin deficiency producing heat aided by yang qi which enters the interior of the body in the afternoon or night and steams yin fluids	Yin deficiency
Tidal fever manifested by a mild sensation of heat in which the skin feels slightly hot when first touched, with the feeling increasing over time. Fever may be aggravated in the afternoon, and combined with heaviness of the head and body	Pathogenic damp which is sticky causing stagnating heat in the interior of the body	Damp warm
Tidal fever manifested by abnormally high body temperature which gradually increases until reaching its highest temperature at 3 to 5 o'clock in the afternoon, then gradually decreasing. May be accompanied by constipation	Excess heat accumulating in yang ming bowels with dry stools in the intestinal tract	Yang ming bowel excess

Mild Fever

Mild fever refers to a body temperature between 99° and 101° F, with the patient having only a slight fever (see Table 4.5).

Table 4.5 Mild Fever

Manifestations	Pathogenesis	Clinical Pattern
Mild fever with spontaneous sweating, mostly occurring in the morning, with poor appetite, listlessness, loose stools	Insufficiency of spleen qi leading to poor promotion of lucid yang	Spleen qi deficiency
Mild fever mostly occurring in the evening, with night sweats, five-palm heat, red zygomatic area	Insufficiency of yin fluids leading to production of deficiency fire	Yin deficiency
Infantile persistent mild fever occurring in summer, thirst, polydipsia, polyuria, light sweating; relieved in autumn	Insufficiency of both qi and yin fluids	Summerheat
Mild fever following late stage warm disease, mostly occurring in the evening	Damp warm retained in the interior of the body	Warm disease

5. ALTERNATING ATTACKS OF FEVER AND CHILLS

Alternating attacks of fever and chills are brought about by pathogens and vital qi fighting each other and mutually advancing and retreating (see Table 4.6).

Table 4.6 Alternating Attacks of Fever and Chills

Manifestations	Pathogenesis	Clinical Pattern
Alternating attacks of fever and chills with irregular onset, bitter taste in mouth, dry throat, dizziness, fullness of the chest and hypochondrium, loss of appetite, wiry pulse	Pathogens entering the half exterior-half interior area of the body where body resistance and pathogens fight each other, manifested by fever if vital qi wins, but chills if pathogens win	Shao yang
Alternating fever and chills with regular onset, severe headache, thirst, and profuse sweating	Pathogens attacking the half exterior-half interior area of the body, manifested by chills if pathogens are entering and struggling against yin, but by high fever as pathogens fight yang to exit	Malaria

II. SWEATING

Sweat is produced by body fluids that are steamed outward by yang qi. Normal sweating can harmonize the ying and wei activities of the body and nourish the skin. Abnormal sweating can be found in many disorders.

Key signs for interrogation

Absence or presence of sweating, time at which sweating occurs, amount of sweat, location of sweating, and main accompanying symptoms are the key signs.

1. ABSENCE OR PRESENCE OF SWEATING

The absence or presence of sweating can help to judge the property of external pathogens, and weakness or prevalence of yang qi in a disorder, particularly in cases of febrile disease.

Presence of Sweating

Presence of sweating can be found in cases of both exterior patterns and interior patterns (see Tables 4.7, 4.8).

Table 4.7 Exterior Pattern with Sweating

Manifestations	Pathogenesis	Clinical Pattern
Mild sweating, aversion to wind, thin white tongue coating, and floating moderate pulse	Wind attacking the surface of the body leading to loosening of the muscular interstices	Exterior deficiency
Sweating, fever greater than chills, sore throat, thin yellow tongue coating, and floating rapid pulse	Wind heat attacking the surface of the body leading to looseness of the muscular interstices	Exterior heat

Table 4.8 Interior Pattern with Sweating

Manifestations	Pathogenesis	Clinical Pattern
Profuse sweating, thirst, fever, flooding pulse	Internal heat stirring and forcing body fluids outward	Interior heat, including qi level and yang ming channel pattern

Absence of Sweating

Absence of sweating can also occur in cases of both exterior patterns and interior patterns (see Tables 4.9, 4.10).

Table 4.9 Exterior Pattern without Sweating

Manifestations	Pathogenesis	Clinical Pattern
Absence of sweating, chills greater than fever, headaches, thin white tongue coating, and floating tense pulse	Wind cold attacking on the surface of the body, leading to tightness of the muscular interstices	Exterior excess

Table 4.10 Interior Pattern without Sweating

Manifestations	Pathogenesis	Clinical Pattern
Absence of sweating, dry skin, severe thirst, scant urine following severe diarrhea, vomiting and other sudden loss of body fluids	Severe impairment of body fluids leading to poor source for sweat	Yin exhaustion
Absence of sweating, cold limbs, aversion to cold, pale face and tongue, tense pulse	Insufficiency of yang qi, or restriction of yang qi by internal cold leading to poor promotion of sweating	Interior cold

2. SPECIAL ASPECTS OF SWEATING

There are several special aspects to note in sweating, including the time at which the sweating occurs, the amount of sweat, and accompanying symptoms (see Table 4.11).

Table 4.11 Special Aspects of Sweating

Manifestations	Pathogenesis	Clinical Pattern
Spontaneous sweating, with listlessness, pale face, and weak pulse; occurring in the daytime and aggravated by exercise	Insufficiency of qi leading to poor tightening of muscular interstices	Qi deficiency
Night sweats, with five-palm heat, red zygomatic area, and thin rapid pulse	Yin deficiency producing heat enhanced by yang qi entering the interior of the body and steaming yin fluids outward	Yin deficiency
Sweating after shivering, seen in febrile diseases	Vital qi and pathogens acutely fighting each other	Exterior

Persistent thick oily sweat, high fever, irritability, severe thirst, thin swift pulse	Collapsed yin fluids going outward	Yin exhaustion
Persistent profuse thin cold sweat, cold limbs, pale face, indistinct pulse	Collapse of yang qi leading to poor consolidation of body fluids	Yang exhaustion

3. LOCALIZED SWEATING

Sweating can occur in different areas of the body according to the etiology and location of an illness (see Tables 4.12 to 4.15).

Table 4.12 Head Sweating

Manifestations	Pathogenesis	Clinical Pattern
Sweating of the head, with red cheeks, thirst, red tongue tip, thin yellow tongue coating, rapid pulse	Abundant heat accumulating in the upper burner and steaming upward	Excess heat
Sweating of the head, with heaviness of the head and even the whole body, discomfort and fullness of the upper abdomen, greasy tongue coating	Damp heat accumulating in the middle burner and steaming upward	Damp heat
Cold sweating on the forehead after chronic and severe illness, shortness of breath, cold limbs, indistinct pulse	Collapse of yang qi following declining yang floating upward	Yang exhaustion

Table 4.13 Unilateral Sweating

Manifestations	Pathogenesis	Clinical Pattern
Sweating on one side of the body, or hemiparalysis with sweating on healthy side of the body	Wind phlegm, wind damp or stagnant blood accumulating in the channels and network vessels	Wind stroke
Sweating only in the upper or lower body, or paraplegia with sweating on upper part of the body	Wind phlegm or blood stasis due to trauma leading to obstruction of the channels and network vessels	Wind stroke; trauma

Table 4.14 Palm and Sole Sweating

Manifestations	Pathogenesis	Clinical Pattern
Profuse sweating in both palms and soles, with dry mouth and throat, five-palm heat, and thin rapid pulse	Insufficiency of yin fluids giving rise to heat and compressing fluids outward	Yin deficiency
Persistent sweating in both palms and soles, with irritability, preference for cold drinks, constipation, dark urine, forceful rapid pulse	Abundant heat accumulating in the yang ming bowel	Yang ming bowel
Sweating in both palms and soles, with heaviness of the head and even the whole body, discomfort and fullness of the upper abdomen, yellow greasy tongue coating	Damp heat steaming outward from the middle burner	Damp heat

Table 4.15 Chest Sweating

Manifestations	Pathogenesis	Clinical Pattern
Chest sweating with listlessness, lassitude, poor appetite, palpitations, loss of sleep	Insufficiency of heart blood combined with insufficiency of spleen qi leading to poor consolidation of heart fluids (sweats)	Heart-spleen deficiency
Chest sweating with palpitations, irritability, dream-disturbed sleep, and soreness and flaccidity of the lumbar area and lower limbs	Insufficiency of kidney yin in the lower body with heart fire flaring upward and compressing heart fluids outwards	Noninteraction of heart and kidney

III. PAIN

Pain is one of most commonly seen symptoms in clinical practice, and may occur in excess, deficiency, heat, or cold patterns. Interrogation about pain should cover the characteristics and duration of pain, location and regularity of occurrence, and accompanying manifestations.

Key Signs for Interrogation

Properties, duration, location of pain, and accompanying manifestations are the key signs.

1. GENERAL PATHOGENESIS OF PAIN

In general, pain is clinically classified into two types. One is caused by an obstruction due to pathogens, and thus a type of excess; the other is due to insufficiency of vital qi, and thus a type of deficiency. General pathogenesis of pain is shown in Table 4.16.

Table 4.16 General Pathogenesis of Pain

Manifestations	Pathogenesis	Clinical Pattern
Pain due to obstruction	Any material pathogens such as blood clots, urinary stones, or food stagnation, leading to qi stagnation and blood stasis obstructing the bowels	Excess
Pain due to poor supplementation	Insufficiency of qi and yang leading to poor warmth; or insufficiency of blood and yin, resulting in poor nourishment	Deficiency

2. PROPERTIES OF PAIN

Pain with different properties arises from different causes (see Table 4.17). Knowing the causes of pain is always the key to the treatment.

Table 4.17 Properties of Pain

Manifestations	Pathogenesis	Clinical Pattern
Distending pain in the chest, upper and lower abdomen	Qi stagnating in the interior of the body	Qi stagnation
Distending pain in the head	Liver qi reversal, liver fire stirring upward, or liver yang rising leading to qi and blood rushing upward	Liver qi reversal, liver fire rising, or liver yang rising
Stabbing pain	Blood stagnating in the channels and network vessels	Blood stasis
Migrating pain	Stagnation of the flow of qi in the channels and network vessels	Qi stagnation
Fixed pain	Stagnation of the flow of blood in the channels and network vessels	Blood stasis
Gripping pain	Material pathogens like parasites, calculi, or blood clots obstructing the flow of qi	Qi stagnation-blood stasis

Radiating pain	Obstruction of the flow of qi	Qi stagnation
Vague pain	Insufficiency of qi, blood, yin, or yang leading to poor nourishment or promotion of blood circulation	Deficiency
Hollow pain	Insufficiency of qi, blood, essence and marrow leading to poor nourishment	Deficiency
Pain with cold sensation	Cold entering and accumulating in the internal organs, the channels, and network vessels	Excess cold
	Insufficiency of yang leading to poor warmth of the internal organs, channels, and network vessels	Deficiency cold
Pain with burning sensation	Excess fire burning the network vessels	Excess heat
	Insufficiency of yin fluids producing deficiency fire burning the network vessels	Deficiency heat
Pain with heavy down-bearing sensation	Damp obstructing the flow of qi and blood	Damp impediment

3. DURATION OF PAIN

This section will compare pain of different duration, or occurring at different times, as these conditions often determine the excess or deficiency properties of the pattern (see Table 4.18).

Table 4.18 Duration of Pain

Manifestations	Pathogenesis	Clinical Pattern
Pain of recent onset	Invasion of external pathogens, trauma	Excess
Chronic pain	Insufficiency of qi, blood or yang	Deficiency
	Obstruction of blood circulation	Blood stasis
Pain aggravated at night	Prosperity of yin, disorders occurring in the blood level	Yin
Pain aggravated in daytime	Prosperity of yang, disorders occurring in the qi level	Yang

Pain with empty stomach	Insufficiency of yang qi leading to poor promotion of the flow of qi and blood	Deficiency
Pain aggravated after food intake	Stagnation of blood and qi leading to obstruction	Excess
Pain before menstruation	Stagnated liver qi accumulating in the chong and ren channels	Qi stagnation
Pain during menstruation	Excess cold attacking the chong and ren channels	Excess cold
	Blood stagnating in the chong and ren channels	Blood stasis
Pain after menstruation	Insufficiency of blood leading to poor nourishment of the chong and ren channels	Blood deficiency

4. LOCATION OF PAIN

In TCM theory, each part of the body is closely related to a certain internal organ or a channel, so the original location of an illness can be determined by asking about the location at which the pain is occurring.

Headache

Headaches may result from external factors, including invasion of wind cold, summer-heat, damp, dryness and fire, or from internal factors, including insufficiency of qi, blood, and essence, phlegm or blood stasis, and dysfunction of the internal organs (see Table 4.19).

Table 4.19 Headaches

Manifestations	Pathogenesis	Clinical Pattern
Sudden, severe, and persistent headache	External wind cold attacking and flaring upward	Exterior excess
Headache radiating to the upper back aggravated by wind	Invasion of external wind leading to stagnation of qi and blood in the upper back	Exterior deficiency
Headache, sore throat, fever, thin yellow tongue coating, floating rapid pulse	External wind heat attacking and stirring upward	Exterior heat

Headache with a sensation of heaviness of the head, limbs, and the whole body	External wind damp attacking and stirring upward	Wind damp
Headache with distending sensation of the head, irritability, malar flush and bloodshot eyes	Liver yang rising, liver qi reversal, liver fire flaring upward leading to qi and blood rushing upwards	Liver yang rising; liver fire flaring upward; liver qi reversal
Vague headache with dizziness, pale lips and face, blurred vision with floaters, pale tongue, and thin pulse	Insufficiency of blood leading to poor nourishment of the head	Blood deficiency
Headache with hollow sensation, soreness and flaccidity of the lumbar area and limbs	Insufficiency of kidney essence leading to poor filling of the sea of marrow	Kidney deficiency
Headache occurring in the forehead	Pathogens attacking the yang ming channel	Yang ming headache
Headache occurring in the posterior of the head	Pathogens attacking the tai yang channel	Tai yang headache
Headache occurring in the temples	Pathogens attacking the shao yang channel	Shao yang headache
Headache occurring in the top of the head	Pathogens attacking the jue yin channel	Jue yin headache

Chest Pain

Pain occurring in the chest is generally related to lung disorders, while pain happening in the precordial area usually indicates a heart disorder (see Table 4.20).

Table 4.20 Chest Pain

Manifestations	Pathogenesis	Clinical Pattern
Left side chest distension; stabbing pain radiating to the left shoulder, arm, and even left upper back	Heart yang qi deficiency leading to poor promotion of qi and blood in the heart vessel; turbid phlegm accumulating in the heart vessel; excess cold accumulating in the heart vessel; qi stagnation leading to blood stasis in the heart vessel	Heart blood stasis

Severe pain in the chest radiating to the back, sudden pale face, cold sweats and cold limbs, loss of consciousness	Sudden collapse of heart yang leading to blockage of the heart vessel	Heart yang exhaustion
Chest pain with high fever, malar flush, cough, asthma, and even flaring of nostrils; occurring in acute respiratory conditions	Excess heat accumulating in the lung	Lung heat
Chest pain with tidal fever, night sweats, red zygomatic area, five-palm heat and bloody sputum; occurring in chronic respiratory conditions	Insufficiency of lung yin leading to upward flaring of deficiency fire	Lung yin deficiency
Distending pain in the chest, coughing, asthma with profuse purulent or bloody sputum; occurring in cases of pulmonary abscess	Toxic heat accumulating in the lung leading to obstruction of qi and blood	Lung heat

Hypochondrial Pain

Hypochondrial pain may occur on one or both sides of the hypochondrium. This symptom is commonly found in liver and gallbladder disorders, because both organs are situated in this area, and the liver and gallbladder channels also circumvent the hypochondrium (see Table 4.21).

Table 4.21 Hypochondrial Pain

Manifestations	Pathogenesis	Clinical Pattern
Distending pain, irritability, frequent sighing	Stagnation of liver qi caused by mental depression	Liver qi stagnation
Burning pain, flushed face, bloodshot eyes, irritability	Excess fire of the liver channel stirring upward	Liver fire
Distending pain, bright yellow skin and sclera, dark urine; occurring in hepatitis A (yang-type jaundice)	Damp heat accumulating in the liver and gallbladder	Liver and gallbladder damp heat
Intercostal distending pain of the affected hypochondrium, aggravated by coughing and deep breathing; occurring in pleurisy	Phlegm fluids retained in the hypochondrium	Phlegm fluids

Distending pain and fullness of hypochondrial area with alternating attacks of fever and chills; occurring in cholecystitis	Pathogens fighting to break down the body's resistance at the half interior-half exterior point of the body	Shao yang

Gastric Pain

Gastric pain is mostly found in stomach disorders from accumulation of cold or heat, retention of food, or qi stagnation, thus leading to reversal of stomach qi (see Table 4.22).

Table 4.22 Gastric Pain

Manifestations	Pathogenesis	Clinical Pattern
Sudden and severe pain relieved by warmth	Excess cold impairing stomach yang	Stomach cold
Burning pain accompanied by hyperactive appetite, bad breath, gum bleeding, and constipation	Fire accumulating in the stomach	Stomach fire
Distending pain with frequent hiccups, aggravated by anger and mental depression; acid reflux	Stagnation of liver qi transversely attacking the stomach	Liver qi attacking the stomach
Vague pain relieved by warmth and pressure, thin saliva	Insufficiency of stomach yang leading to poor warmth of the stomach	Stomach yang deficiency
Burning pain, discomfort, hunger with no desire for food, red tongue with scant coating	Insufficiency of stomach yin leading to production of deficiency fire	Stomach yin deficiency

Abdominal Pain

In TCM, the abdomen is generally divided into the upper abdomen and the lower abdomen, with the umbilicus as the dividing line. Pain in the upper abdomen is closely related to spleen and stomach disorders, while pain in the lower abdomen is related to the disorders occurring in the kidney, bladder, large intestine, and small intestine. Pain caused by an accumulation of cold, heat, or parasites, or a stagnation of qi, blood, or food indicates excess patterns; pain due to an insufficiency of qi, blood, and yang indicates deficiency patterns (see Table 4.23).

Table 4.23 Abdominal Pain

Manifestations	Pathogenesis	Clinical Pattern
Vague pain relieved by warmth and pressure	Insufficiency of qi, blood, yin, or yang	Deficiency
Severe pain aggravated by pressure	Accumulation of heat, cold, parasites, or calculi, or stagnation of qi, blood, or food	Excess

Lumbar Pain

Lumbar pain is mainly caused by kidney deficiency or an accumulation of cold damp in the lower back. Lumbar pain due to qi and blood stagnation is always associated with trauma (see Table 4.24).

Table 4.24 Lumbar Pain

Manifestations	Pathogenesis	Clinical Pattern
Vague and persistent pain with soreness and flaccidity of the lumbar area; aggravated by exercise, relieved by resting	Insufficiency of kidney leading to poor nourishment of the lumbar area	Kidney deficiency
Pain with downbearing sensation of the lumbosacral area; aggravated by bad weather, relieved by heat	Invasion of cold damp disturbing qi and blood flow	Cold damp
Pain with limited range of motion and aggravated at night; trauma history	Qi and blood stagnation leading to blockage of channels and network vessels	Qi stagnation and blood stasis

Pain in the Limbs

Pain in the limbs refers to pain occurring in the joints, bones, muscles, and tendons of the limbs. It is commonly found in impediment patterns caused by wind, cold, and dampness attacking individually or in combination with each other (see Table 4.25). However, sometimes an impediment pattern may be caused by kidney deficiency.

Table 4.25 Pain in the Limbs

Manifestations	Pathogenesis	Clinical Pattern
Migrating pain in the joints	External wind attacking the joints leading to stagnation of qi and blood	Wind impediment
Severe pain in the joints with spasms of the muscles; relieved by warmth	Wind cold attacking the joints leading to stagnation of qi and blood	Cold impediment
Pain in the joint marked by sensation of heaviness in the affected limb	Damp invading and retained in the joint leading to stagnation of qi and blood	Damp impediment
Pain in the joint, redness, swelling, and sensation of heat in the affected area	Wind heat attacking the joint leading to stagnation of qi and blood	Heat impediment
Pain of the heel and shin; with flaccidity of the lower limbs, soreness of the lumbar area	Weakness of kidney leading to poor nourishment of the limbs	Kidney deficiency

Aching

Aching refers to pain or generalized discomfort of the whole body. The onset type is the key to the identification of its clinical pattern (see Table 4.26).

Table 4.26 Aching

Manifestations	Pathogenesis	Clinical Pattern
Severe aching of recent onset, accompanied by chills and fever	Invasion of wind, cold, and damp leading to obstruction of qi and blood in the channels and network vessels	Exterior
Persistent mild aching seen in chronic cases, listlessness; relieved by resting	Deficiency of qi, blood, yin, and yang bringing about poor warmth and nourishment of the body	Deficiency

IV. OTHER DISORDERS OF THE HEAD, BODY, CHEST, AND ABDOMEN

Other than pain, various abnormal feelings may occur in the head, chest, abdomen, and possibly the entire body. These will be examined in this section.

Key Signs for Interrogation

Severity and characteristics of each abnormal sensation.

1. DIZZINESS

Dizziness may be mild, with the patient feeling some giddiness, or severe, to the point where the patient has the sense of both his body and the environment revolving around him and is unable to stand steadily. During interrogation, special attention should be given to predisposing causes and other factors that aggravate the dizziness (see Table 4.27).

Table 4.27 Dizziness

Manifestations	Pathogenesis	Clinical Pattern
Dizziness with pale complexion, palpitations, insomnia, numbness of extremities, pale face, listlessness, lassitude; aggravated by exercise	Insufficiency of qi and blood leading to poor nourishment of the brain	Qi-blood deficiency
Dizziness with soreness of the lumbar area, lassitude, tinnitus, nocturnal emissions, and five-palm heat	Insufficiency of kidney essence leading to poor support of the marrow	Kidney essence deficiency
Dizziness, with headaches, irritability, bitter taste, malar flush, bloodshot eyes, red tongue, wiry rapid pulse	Excess heat of the liver channel flaring upward	Liver fire rising
Dizziness, with distending pain of the head, tinnitus, soreness and weakness of the lumbar area and knees, wiry thin pulse	Insufficiency of kidney and liver yin in the lower half of the body with rising of liver yang in the upper body	Liver yang rising
Dizziness with sensation of heaviness and whirling in the head, nausea, vomiting, white greasy tongue coating	Accumulation of phlegm damp leading to poor promotion of lucid yang	Phlegm
Dizziness with stabbing pain of the head following trauma	Stagnation of qi and obstruction of blood	Blood stasis

2. OPPRESSION OF THE CHEST

Oppression of the chest refers to a condition of distension and fullness with pressure on the chest. It is closely related to stagnation of lung and heart qi (see Table 4.28).

Table 4.28 Oppression of the Chest

Manifestations	Pathogenesis	Clinical Pattern
Oppression of the chest with palpitations, shortness of breath	Insufficiency of heart qi and yang leading to poor promotion of heart blood	Heart yang qi deficiency
Oppression of the chest with stabbing pain	Stagnation of blood and qi occurring in the heart vessel	Heart blood stasis
Oppression of the chest with coughing, asthma, and possibly profuse sputum	Phlegm damp disturbing the chest leading to stagnation of lung qi	Phlegm

3. PALPITATIONS

Palpitations are a symptom marked by a flustered, unsettled feeling that is uncontrollable and accompanied by a rapid heartbeat. Palpitations occur in almost all heart disorders (see Table 4.29).

Table 4.29 Palpitations

Manifestations	Pathogenesis	Clinical Pattern
Palpitations, with pale face, shortness of breath, lassitude, spontaneous sweating, weak pulse	Insufficiency of heart qi resulting in poor promotion of blood circulation	Heart qi deficiency
Palpitations, with pale face, aversion to cold, cold limbs, listlessness, pale tongue, and deep slow pulse	Insufficiency of heart yang leading to poor promotion of blood circulation	Heart yang deficiency
Palpitations with pale face, lips, and nails, pale tongue, thin pulse	Insufficiency of heart blood leading to poor filling of blood vessels	Heart blood deficiency
Palpitations, with red zygomatic area, night sweats, irritability and five-palm heat, scant tongue coating, and thin rapid pulse	Insufficiency of heart yin resulting in production of deficiency heat	Heart yin deficiency
Severe palpitations, sudden paleness of the face, cold limbs, cold sweat, and feeble pulse	Sudden collapse of heart yang leading to sudden decline of warmth and promotion of the heart	Yang exhaustion

Sudden palpitations with pain in the chest radiating to the back, purple tongue, and choppy pulse	Obstruction of heart vessels leading to poor nourishment of the heart	Heart blood stasis
Severe palpitations occurring in the xiphoid region with pale face, cold limbs, general edema	Retention of body fluids leading to water qi attacking the heart	Water qi attacking the heart
Palpitations due to fright	Stirring up of phlegm heat and stagnation of gallbladder qi	Gallbladder depression-phlegm fire stirring upward

4. DISTENSION OF THE HYPOCHONDRIUM

Distension can occur on one or both sides of the hypochondrium. It is commonly related to liver and gallbladder disorders (see Table 4.30).

Table 4.30 Distension of the Hypochondrium

Manifestations	Pathogenesis	Clinical Pattern
Distension and discomfort of the hypochondrium, irritability, frequent sighing	Emotional depression leading to stagnation of liver qi	Liver qi stagnation
Distension of the hypochondrium, bitter taste in mouth, nausea, yellow greasy tongue coating	Damp heat accumulating in the liver and gallbladder leading to stagnation of liver qi	Liver-gallbladder damp heat

5. FULLNESS OF THE UPPER ABDOMEN

Fullness of the upper abdomen refers to an uncomfortable feeling of oppression and distension in the gastric area (see Table 4.31).

Table 4.31 Fullness of the Upper Abdomen

Manifestations	Pathogenesis	Clinical Pattern
Fullness and discomfort of the upper abdomen, tenderness, belching, acid reflux, dyspepsia, rolling pulse	Improper food intake impairing the spleen and stomach and leading to poor digestion	Food stagnation
Fullness and discomfort of the upper abdomen, relieved by pressure, poor appetite, loose stools, weak pulse	Weakness of the spleen and stomach leading to dysfunction in transportation and transformation	Spleen deficiency

6. DISTENSION OF THE ABDOMEN

Distension of the abdomen refers to a sense of enlargement and tightness of the abdomen, like a full balloon. When tapping the abdomen, it has a drum-like sound (see Table 4.32).

Table 4.32 Distension of the Upper Abdomen

Manifestations	Pathogenesis	Clinical Pattern
Distension of the abdomen which is relieved by pressure, poor appetite, loose stools, weak pulse	Weakness of the spleen and stomach	Deficiency
Distension and tenderness of the abdomen, wiry rolling pulse	Excess heat and food accumulating in the intestinal tract obstructing the flow of qi	Excess
Distension with enlarged abdomen; ascites occurring in late-staged hepatic diseases	Indulgence in alcohol and/or emotional stress impairing the function of the liver, spleen, and kidney leading to qi and blood stagnation and body fluids accumulating in the abdomen	Accumulation

7. HEAVINESS OF THE BODY

Heaviness of the body refers to an uncomfortable feeling in the whole body, marked by soreness and lassitude with no interest in exercise. It is closely related to lung and spleen disorders (see Table 4.33).

Table 4.33 Heaviness of the Body

Manifestations	Pathogenesis	Clinical Pattern
Heaviness of the body, even edema starting with the eyelids, the face, and then the whole body; floating pulse	Invasion of external wind leading to failure of the lung to dredge the water passages	Wind water attacking the lung
Heaviness of the body, lassitude, listlessness, shortness of breath, poor appetite, weak pulse	Insufficiency of spleen qi leading to failure of the spleen to transport damp	Spleen deficiency

8. NUMBNESS OF THE BODY

Numbness refers to having little or no sensation in the skin (see Table 4.34).

Table 4.34 Numbness of the Body

Manifestations	Pathogenesis	Clinical Pattern
Numbness, with pale face and lips, lassitude, palpitations, poor appetite, weak thin pulse	Insufficiency of both qi and blood leading to poor promotion of blood flow and nourishment of the body	Qi-blood deficiency
Numbness of the body, aching, limited range of motion in the joints, hemiparesis	Damp phlegm or blood stasis obstructing the channels and network vessels	Wind stroke

V. Ears and Eyes

The ears are the opening of the kidney, while the eyes are the opening of the liver. Therefore, symptoms occurring in the ears and eyes help to identify disorders related to the liver and kidney.

1. Ears

Tinnitus, deafness, and auditory suppression are the most common disorders of the ears. Tinnitus and deafness can occur singly or in combination. Auditory suppression and deafness are often a result of tinnitus.

Tinnitus

Tinnitus refers to a continuous sound in the ears like a cicada or a tide coming in. To some extent, it affects hearing (see Table 4.35).

Table 4.35 Tinnitus

Manifestations	Pathogenesis	Clinical Pattern
Sudden tinnitus like a tidal surge, not relieved by pressure on the ears	Stirring of liver-gallbladder fire leading to obstruction of hearing	Excess
Tinnitus like the sound of cicadas, occuring gradually following a chronic illness process or in cases of poor constitution	Liver yin-kidney yin deficiency leading to liver yang rising; kidney essence deficiency leading to poor filling of the sea of marrow (brain)	Deficiency

Deafness

A sudden onset of deafness indicates an excess pattern and is comparatively easy to heal, but chronic deafness is found in deficiency patterns and is hard to cure (see Table 4.36).

Table 4.36 Deafness

Manifestations	Pathogenesis	Clinical Pattern
Sudden deafness	Stirring upward of liver-gallbladder fire leading to obstruction of the hearing	Excess
Gradual deafness	Insufficiency of kidney qi leading to poor promotion of hearing	Deficiency

Auditory Suppression

Auditory suppression refers to weakness of hearing with repeated echoes (see Table 4.37).

Table 4.37 Auditory Suppression

Manifestations	Pathogenesis	Clinical Pattern
Sudden auditory suppression	Stirring of external wind or turbid phlegm leading to obstruction of hearing	Excess
Gradual auditory suppression	Insufficiency of kidney essence qi leading to poor promotion and nourishment of hearing	Deficiency

2. EYES

Most disorders of the eyes have been discussed in Chapter Two above, so only a few symptoms will be mentioned in this section.

Itching

This refers to itching occurring in the eyelids, canthi, and eyeballs (see Table 4.38).

Table 4.38 Itching

Manifestations	Pathogenesis	Clinical Pattern
With acute onset, itching of the eyelid, canthus, and eyeball as from a creeping insect, tearing in bright sunlight, burning sensation	Stirring upward of wind heat from the liver channel	Excess
With chronic mild itching, pale lips and face, thin pulse	Insufficiency of liver blood leading to poor nourishment of the eyes	Deficiency

Pain

Eye pain can occur in one or both eyes. Severe pain is usually seen in excess patterns and mild pain in deficiency patterns. Excess patterns with pain in the eyes are more commonly found in clinical practice (see Table 4.39).

Table 4.39 Pain

Manifestations	Pathogenesis	Clinical Pattern
Severe pain of the eyes, flushed face, bloodshot eyes, bitter taste in mouth, irritability	Excess fire of the liver channel flaring upward	Excess
Pain and swelling of the eyelids, severely bloodshot eyes, photophobia, gumminess of the eyes	External wind heat attacking and flaring upward	Exterior
Mild pain always occurring in the evening, dryness and discomfort of the eyeball, five-palm heat, night sweats, thin rapid pulse	Insufficiency of liver-kidney yin causing stirring of deficiency fire	Yin deficiency

Dim Eyesight

Dim eyesight refers to a symptom marked by blurred vision with floaters affecting the visual field (see Table 4.40).

Table 4.40 Dim Eyesight

Manifestations	Pathogenesis	Clinical Pattern
Dim eyesight, flushed face, distension of the head, headache	Wind fire flaring upward and stirring in the orifices	Excess heat
Dim eyesight, mental confusion, fuzzy thoughts, heaviness of the head and body, nausea and poor appetite	Turbid phlegm stirring in and restricting the orifices	Phlegm
Dim eyesight, lassitude and listlessness, shortness of breath, dizziness, weak pulse occurring in the old and in chronic cases	Spleen qi deficiency leading to sinking of lucid yang	Qi sinking
Dim eyesight, soreness and flaccidity of the lumbar area and knees, tinnitus, dizziness, night sweats, low-grade fever, rapid thin pulse occurring in the weak, the old, and in chronic cases	Liver and kidney yin deficiency leading to poor nourishment of the eyes	Liver-kidney yin deficiency

Other Abnormalities of Vision

Other abnormalities of vision include blurred vision, night blindness, color blindness, and double vision, all of which are most commonly found in the weak, the old, and in lingering cases, and are caused by insufficiency of liver blood and kidney essence leading to poor nourishment of the eyes.

VI. SLEEP

Regular sleep helps one adapt to the regular changes of day and night in nature, and keeps the body's yin and yang in balance. In a normal healthy state, wei qi circulates through the yang channels during the daytime, allowing excess yang qi to keep the body awake. At night, wei qi travels through the yin channels, and the excess of yin qi therefore allows the body to sleep. Besides its function in harmonizing yin and yang, sleep is also related to the prevalence or insufficiency of qi and blood, as well as the function of the heart and kidney. Abnormal sleep is clinically classified into insomnia and somnolence.

Key Signs for Interrogation

Duration of sleep, ability to fall asleep, dream-disturbed sleep.

1. INSOMNIA

Insomnia is generally caused by yang qi failing to enter the yin system, and the mind failing to become calm (see Table 4.41).

Table 4.41 Insomnia

Manifestations	Pathogenesis	Clinical Pattern
Difficulty falling asleep, irritability, dream-disturbed sleep, tidal fever, night sweats, and soreness and flaccidity of the loin and knees	Insufficiency of kidney yin (water) in the lower body with stirring upward of heart fire	Noninteraction of heart and kidney
Easily awakened earlier in the morning, hyperactive mind, poor appetite, loose stools, listlessness, pale tongue, and weak pulse	Deficiency of spleen qi providing a poor source for qi and blood, accompanied by insufficiency of heart blood leading to poor nourishment of the mind	Heart-spleen deficiency
Easily awakened, dream-disturbed sleep, palpitations due to fright, timidity, hesitation, irritability, bitter taste in mouth, and nausea	Stirring of phlegm heat accompanied by stagnation of gallbladder qi	Gallbladder depression–phlegm fire stirring upward

| Insomnia, restlessness, fullness and distension of the upper abdomen, acid reflux, and thick greasy tongue coating | Improper food intake leading to reversal of stomach qi | Food stagnation |

2. SOMNOLENCE

Somnolence refers to a condition in which the patient always feels sleepy and easily falls asleep (see Table 4.42).

Table 4.42 Somnolence

Manifestations	Pathogenesis	Clinical Pattern
Sleepiness, fuzzy thoughts, with listlessness, dizziness, fullness of the upper abdomen, heavy sensation of the whole body and head, greasy tongue coating, and soft pulse	Phlegm damp disturbing the spleen leading to failure of lucid yang to rise	Phlegm damp
Sleepiness aggravated by food intake, listlessness, lassitude, poor appetite, and weak pulse	Spleen qi deficiency leading to failure of lucid yang to rise	Spleen qi deficiency
Sleepiness, severe listlessness, and even fuzzy thoughts, cold limbs, and feeble pulse	Heart-kidney yang deficiency leading to collapse of organ function	Heart-kidney yang deficiency
Sleepiness, with high fever, delirium aggravated at night, mental confusion, macules and papules	Heat penetrating the pericardium	Ying level, blood level

VII. THIRST, APPETITE, AND TASTE

Many disorders will affect food and drink intake, as food and drink are the source of acquired essence and qi, on which all biological activities depend. Through interrogation about food intake, the prevalence or insufficiency of body fluids and the current state of the spleen, stomach, and other organs related to digestion can be learned.

Key Signs for Interrogation

Thirst, food intake, and taste are the key signs.

1. ABSENCE OF THIRST AND PRESENCE OF THIRST

The absence or presence of thirst reflects the metabolic condition of the body fluids.

Absence of Thirst with No Desire to Drink

An absence of thirst with no desire to drink shows that body fluids have not been impaired. It is commonly seen in cold patterns and damp patterns (see Table 4.43).

Table 4.43 Absence of Thirst

Manifestations	Pathogenesis	Clinical Pattern
Absence of thirst, aversion to cold, cold limbs	Cold accumulating in the interior of the body	Cold
Absence of thirst, heaviness of the body, tooth-marks on the tongue, soft pulse	Damp accumulating in the interior of the body	Damp

Presence of Thirst with Desire to Drink

Presence of thirst with desire to drink shows that body fluids have been impaired. It is commonly seen in heat patterns and dryness patterns (see Table 4.44).

Table 4.44 Presence of Thirst

Manifestations	Pathogenesis	Clinical Pattern
Severe thirst with desire to drink, malar flush, profuse sweating, fever, flooding pulse	Abundant heat stagnating in the interior of the body	Excess heat
Severe thirst, polyuria, hyperactive appetite and emaciation; occurring in diabetes	Insufficiency of kidney qi and yin leading to dysfunction of water metabolism	Qi and yin deficiency
Thirst following severe diarrhea, vomiting, and profuse sweating	Impairment of body fluids	Yin deficiency

Thirst Without Desire to Drink

Thirst without an accompanying desire to drink is usually caused by failure of qi to steam upwards and distribute body fluids (see Table 4.45).

Diagnosis in Traditional Chinese Medicine

Table 4.45 Thirst without Desire to Drink

Manifestations	Pathogenesis	Clinical Pattern
Thirst with tidal fever, night sweats, flushed zygomatic region, and five-palm heat	Warm pathogen retained at the ying level and streaming ying fluid upward	Ying level
Thirst, with heavy sensation of the head and the whole body, fullness of the upper abdomen, and greasy tongue coating	Damp heat accumulating in the interior of the body and steaming upward	Damp heat
Thirst, dizziness, splashing sound in the upper abdomen, drooling	Phlegm fluids retained in the stomach	Phlegm fluids
Thirst with stabbing pain following traumatic injury, purple tongue, and choppy pulse	Blood stagnating in the interior of the body leading to failure in the distribution of body fluids	Blood stasis

2. APPETITE

Good appetite refers to both the need and the pleasurable desire to eat. Disorders occurring in the spleen, stomach, and other organs that are related to digestion commonly give rise to abnormal appetite.

Poor Appetite

Poor appetite means lack of interest in eating, a feeling of discomfort after a small amount of food intake, or having a poor appetite (see Table 4.46).

Table 4.46 Poor Appetite

Manifestations	Pathogenesis	Clinical Pattern
Poor appetite with emaciation, distension of the abdomen, diarrhea, pale tongue, and weak pulse	Insufficiency of spleen qi leading to poor promotion of digestion	Spleen qi deficiency
Poor appetite with fullness of upper abdomen, heavy sensation of the head and the whole body, loose stools, tooth marks on the tongue, greasy tongue coating	Damp disturbance in the spleen leading to poor transportation and transformation	Damp disturbing the spleen

Poor appetite with dislike of greasy foods, jaundice, painful hypochondrium	Accumulation of damp heat in the liver and gallbladder	Damp heat
Discomfort after small amount of food intake, with distending pain of the abdomen, tenderness, acid reflux, hiccups, and greasy tongue coating following improper food intake	Undigested food stagnating in the stomach leading to reversal of stomach qi	Food stagnation
Poor appetite seen in pregnant women, morning sickness, rolling pulse occurring in pregnancy, vomiting	Reversal of qi from the chong vessel leading to reversal of stomach qi	Stomach qi reversal

Hyperactive Appetite

Hyperactive appetite refers to a condition in which the appetite is greater than normal, but in which hunger is easily induced and the digestion is not always severely affected (see Table 4.47).

Table 4.47 Hyperactive Appetite

Manifestations	Pathogenesis	Clinical Pattern
Hyperactive appetite with thirst, irritability, bad breath, constipation, gum bleeding, red tongue with yellow coating	Upward stirring of stomach fire leading to hyperfunction of digestion	Stomach fire
Hyperactive appetite with loose stools containing undigested food, emaciation, pale face and tongue	Hyperactive stomach receives too much food which a weak spleen is unable to transport and transform	Hyperactivity of the stomach–weakness of the spleen

Other Abnormalities in Appetite

See Table 4.48.

Table 4.48 Other Abnormalities in Appetite

Manifestations	Pathogenesis	Clinical Pattern
Hunger with no desire for food because of discomfort in the gastric area after meals, dry mouth and throat, red tongue with scant coating, rapid thin pulse	Insufficiency of stomach yin leading to poor nourishment of the stomach and stirring of deficiency fire	Stomach yin deficiency

Emaciation, malnutrition with strong desire to eat clay, raw rice, and other unusual things; particularly occurring in parasitosis in infants	Parasites accumulating in the intestines leading to dysfunction of the spleen in transformation and transportation	Spleen deficiency

3. TASTE

The mouth is the opening of the spleen. Abnormal tastes are commonly found in disorders occurring in the spleen and other organs that aid in digestion (see Table 4.49).

Table 4.49 Abnormal Tastes

Manifestations	Pathogenesis	Clinical Pattern
Loss of taste, poor appetite, loose stools, distension of the abdomen	Insufficiency of stomach and spleen qi leading to poor promotion of digestion	Spleen qi-stomach qi deficiency
Sweet taste with sticky and greasy sensation, poor appetite, fullness of the upper abdomen	Damp heat accumulating in the stomach and spleen and steaming upward	Spleen-stomach damp heat
Sour taste, abdominal pain, acid reflux, frequent belching, emotional depression	Stagnation of liver qi transversely attacking the stomach	Disharmony between liver and stomach
Sour taste, bad breath, distension of the upper abdomen, hiccups following improper food intake	Undigested food stagnating in the stomach leading to production of heat	Food stagnation
Bitter taste in mouth, hypochondriac pain, irritabililty, red eyes,wiry pulse	Abundance of liver-gallbladder fire leading to reversal of gallbladder qi	Liver-gallbladder fire
Salty taste, low back pain, weak knees	Insufficiency of kidney qi leading to an upsurge of cold water	Kidney deficiency

VIII. DEFECATION AND URINATION

Defecation and urination are related to digestion and the metabolism of body fluids.

Key Signs for Interrogation

Character, color, odor, and amount of stools and urine, or degree of difficulty in defecation and urination are the key signs.

1. DEFECATION

Defecation is affected by the functions of the spleen and stomach in transforming and transporting, of the liver and gallbladder in dispersing, of the life gate in warming and promoting, and of the lung in moving downward.

Constipation

Constipation refers to defecation with difficulty. Generally, this is due to dry stools, but there can be chronic cases where the stools may be either dry or soft (see Table 4.50).

Table 4.50 Constipation

Manifestations	Pathogenesis	Clinical Pattern
Dry stools with difficult defecation, irritability, fever, thirst, scant and dry urine, rolling rapid pulse	Excess heat impairing body fluids leading to dryness of the intestinal tract	Excess heat
Dry stools with abdominal pain, high fever or tidal fever aggravated in the afternoon, abdominal tenderness, pulse with strong beat	Heat accumulating in the intestinal tract with dry stools	Yang ming bowel
Defecation with difficulty; occurring in chronic cases, the old, postpartum, or in patients with constitutional weakness	Insufficiency of qi, blood, and body fluids leading to poor moistening and promotion of defecation	Deficiency
Constipation with abdominal pain aggravated by pressure but relieved by warmth; cold limbs and pale face, deep slow pulse	Excess cold accumulating in the intestinal tract	Excess cold

Diarrhea

Diarrhea refers to frequent defecation with poorly formed and possibly watery stools (see Table 4.51).

Table 4.51 Diarrhea

Manifestations	Pathogenesis	Clinical Pattern
Loose stools, even watery stools containing undigested food, poor appetite, distension of the abdomen	Insufficiency of spleen qi leading to dysfunction in transformation	Spleen qi deficiency

Manifestations	Pathogenesis	Clinical Pattern
Diarrhea before dawn, aversion to cold, cold limbs, soreness and weakness in the loin and knees, vague pain of the abdomen relieved by defecation	Insufficiency of kidney-spleen yang leading to life gate fire failing to generate earth (spleen)	Spleen-kidney yang deficiency
Diarrhea alternating with dry stools, with abdominal pain following anger or emotional depression; anal burning and discomfort during defecation	Stagnated liver qi attacking the spleen leading to dysfunction in transformation and transportation	Disharmony between liver and spleen
Diarrhea with sticky and yellow stools, anal burning and discomfort during defecation, loss of appetite	Damp heat accumulating in the intestinal tract and disturbing the flow of qi	Spleen-stomach damp heat
Diarrhea followed by abdominal pain, purulent and bloody stools, tenesmus, and history of unclean food intake	Damp heat disturbing the intestinal tract and damaging the blood vessels	Large intestine damp heat
Loose stools with foul smell, loss of appetite, distension and fullness of the abdomen, acid reflux, or anal discomfort during defecation	Undigested food accumulating in the intestinal tract	Food stagnation

Abnormal Sensation during Defecation

Abnormal sensation in defecation refers to any abnormal feeling around the anus or possibly in the abdomen (see Table 4.52).

Table 4.52 Abnormal Sensation During Defecation

Manifestations	Pathogenesis	Clinical Pattern
Anal burning sensation	Downward flow of damp heat from the large intestine	Large intestine damp heat
Tenesmus	Damp heat disturbing the large intestine leading to qi stagnation	Large intestine damp heat
Anal discomfort during defecation, yellow, thick stools containing partially digested fat	Damp heat accumulating in the large intestine leading to qi stagnation	Spleen-stomach damp heat; disharmony between the liver and spleen
Anal discomfort during defecation, abdominal pain and distension, diarrhea, emotional depression	Liver qi stagnating and attacking the spleen	Liver qi stagnation

Anal discomfort during defecation with improper food intake, fullness of upper abdomen, and acid reflux	Undigested food retained in the stomach producing damp heat	Food stagnation
Fecal incontinence occurring in lingering severe illnesses or the old	Insufficiency of kidney qi leading to loss of control of the anus	Kidney qi deficiency
Downbearing sensation in the anus, collapse of the rectum following defecation, aggravated by doing manual labor	Extreme spleen qi deficiency leading to poor promotion of the internal organs	Sinking of spleen qi

2. URINATION

Urination is directly governed by the bladder. In addition, it is also affected by the function of the kidney in promoting functional bladder qi, the spleen in transporting body fluids, the lung in moving qi downward and to the triple burner in draining water passages.

Abnormal Frequency of Urination

The abnormal frequency of urination includes the conditions of frequent or difficult urination, and possibly retention of urine (see Table 4.53).

Table 4.53 Abnormal Frequency of Urination

Manifestations	Pathogenesis	Clinical Pattern
Frequent urination, painful urgent urination and scant and dark urine, burning sensation during urination	Damp heat accumulating in the lower burner	Bladder damp heat
Frequent urination often occurring at night, clear urine in large amounts, even incontinence of urine	Insufficiency of kidney qi leading to dysfunction in opening and closing of the bladder	Kidney qi deficiency
Difficult urination, possibly retention of the urine, distending pain of the lower abdomen, abdominal tenderness; occurring in cases of urinary stones, bladder cancer, or severe UTI (urinary tract infection)	Qi and blood stagnation, obstruction by calculus or damp heat accumulating in the lower burner	Excess
Difficult urination, possibly retention of urine; occurring in the old or in lingering and severe cases such as uremia	Insufficiency of kidney qi leading to dysfunction in opening and closing of the bladder	Deficiency

Abnormal Amount of Urine

Abnormal amount of urine includes excessive or scanty urine (see Table 4.54).

Table 4.54 Abnormal Amount of Urine

Manifestations	Pathogenesis	Clinical Pattern
Clear urine in large amounts, aversion to cold, preference for warmth and pressure	Insufficiency of kidney yang qi leading to dysfunction in opening and closing of the bladder	Deficiency cold
Clear urine in large amounts, polydipsia, polyphagia and emaciation; occurring in diabetes	Insufficiency of lung-kidney qi and yin leading to dysfunction of the bladder in opening and closing	Lung-kidney qi and yin deficiency
Scant and dark urine with fever, thirst, flushed face, sweating, and constipation	Excess heat accumulating inside the body and consuming the body fluids	Excess heat
Scanty urine after profuse sweating, severe vomiting or diarrhea	Consumption of body fluids leading to poor production of urine	Yin deficiency
Scant urine with edema on eyelids, around the ankles and legs	Dysfunction of the lung, spleen, and kidney leading to abnormal metabolism of body fluids	Damp retention

Abnormal Sensations During Urination

Abnormal sensations during urination include painful, urgent, dribbling urination with discomfort of the meatus urinarius, urinary incontinence, and bedwetting (see Table 4.55).

Table 4.55 Abnormal Sensations during Urination

Manifestations	Pathogenesis	Clinical Pattern
Painful, urgent urination with burning sensation	Damp heat accumulating in the lower burner and flowing downward	Bladder damp heat
Dribbling urination occurring in the old, or lingering illnesses, combined with a weak constitution	Insufficiency of kidney qi leading to dysfunction in the opening and closing of the bladder	Kidney qi deficiency
Urinary incontinence, loss of consciousness, soreness and flaccidity of the lumbar area and knees	Insufficiency of kidney qi leading to dysfunction in the opening and closing of the bladder	Kidney qi deficiency

Urinary incontinence, loss of consciousness, usually occurring in emergency and severe cases	Decline of kidney qi leading to poor consolidation of the bladder	Collapse of kidney qi
Bedwetting	Insufficiency of kidney qi leading to dysfunction of the bladder in opening and closing	Kidney qi deficiency

IX. ABNORMAL SEXUAL FUNCTION

Abnormal sexual function is closely related to the functions of the kidney according to Chinese medical theories.

Key Signs for Interrogation

Sexual potency, seminal emission, spermatorrhea, and premature ejaculation.

1. IMPOTENCE

Impotence refers to the inability to perform coitus. Although this is mainly a disorder of males caused by a failure to achieve an erection, it may occur in women due to structural anomalies or painful inflammations with spasms of the muscles around the vagina. These spasms may also be caused by anxiety (see Table 4.56).

Table 4.56 Impotence

Manifestations	Pathogenesis	Clinical Pattern
Impotence following indulgence in sexual activity, emotional distress	Impairment of kidney yin and yang leading to decline of life gate fire causing poor warmth of the body	Kidney yang deficiency
Impotence occurring in the old, the weak, or in lingering cases, listlessness, soreness and weakness of the lumbar area and knees relieved by warmth	Decline of life gate fire leading to poor warmth of the body	Kidney yang deficiency

2. SEMINAL EMISSION

Seminal emission refers to irregular ejaculation occurring outside of sexual activity. It can occur either in the daytime or at night with accompanying dream-disturbed sleep (see Table 4.57).

Table 4.57 Seminal Emission

Manifestations	Pathogenesis	Clinical Pattern
Nocturnal emission following overindulgence in sexual activity, emotional distress, with dizziness, tinnitus, dream-disturbed sleep, irritability, soreness of the lumbar area, and weak knees	Impairment of kidney yin leading to stirring upward of ministerial fire	Kidney yin deficiency
Seminal emission occurring in the old, the weak or in lingering cases, listlessness, aversion to cold, cold limbs	Decline of life gate fire leading to poor warmth	Kidney yang deficiency

3. SPERMATORRHEA

Spermatorrhea refers to irregular seminal emission occurring outside of sexual activity (see Table 4.58).

Table 4.58 Spermatorrhea

Manifestations	Pathogenesis	Clinical Pattern
Spermatorrhea occurring in the old, the weak, and in lingering cases; aversion to cold, lassitude and listlessness, soreness and weakness of the lumbar area and knees relieved by warmth	Insufficiency of kidney yang leading to poor warmth	Kidney yang deficiency
Spermatorrhea with bedwetting, frequent urination or even incontinence of urine, impotence, premature ejaculation occurring in the old or in lingering cases	Insufficiency of kidney qi leading to poor consolidation of sperm	Kidney qi deficiency

4. PREMATURE EJACULATION

Premature ejaculation always occurs in those with yang deficiency, and is frequently found in those who indulge in an excess of sexual activity (see Table 4.59).

Table 4.59 Premature Ejaculation

Manifestations	Pathogenesis	Clinical Pattern
Premature ejaculation, listlessness and lassitude, spermatorrhea, cold limbs, and aversion to cold with a preference for warmth	Insufficiency of kidney yang leading to poor warmth	Kidney yang deficiency

Premature ejaculation, spermatorrhea, frequent urination, or nocturia and incontinence of urine	Insufficiency of kidney qi leading to poor consolidation	Kidney qi deficiency

X. ABNORMAL MENSTRUATION

All women of normal menstrual age should be questioned regarding their menstrual cycle, as this is often related to a other disorders they may be experiencing.

Key Signs for Interrogation

Menstrual cycle, duration of menstruation, as well as amount, color, and thickness of the blood, dysmenorrhea, or amenorrhea are the key signs. In addition, the last menstrual period and the age of menarche or menopause should be determined, as indicated by the patient's condition and age.

1. SHORTENED MENSTRUAL CYCLE

A shortened menstrual cycle lasts 8 days less than the standard length of 28 days between the onsets of two successive periods (see Table 4.60).

Table 4.60 Shortened Menstrual Cycle

Manifestations	Pathogenesis	Clinical Pattern
Excessive menstruation, light-colored thin blood, listlessness, poor appetite, pale face and tongue, weak pulse	Insufficiency of spleen qi leading to failure to keep blood circulating inside the vessels	Spleen qi deficiency
Excessive menstruation, dark-colored and thick blood, irritability, thirst, and even fever; red tongue, rapid pulse	Heat in the blood compressing the blood out of the vessels	Blood heat

2. DELAYED MENSTRUAL CYCLE

A delayed menstrual cycle lasts eight days longer than the standard length of 28 days between the onset of two successive periods (see Table 4.61).

Table 4.61 Delayed Menstrual Cycle

Manifestations	Pathogenesis	Clinical Pattern
Scant menstruation, light-colored and thin vaginal blood, dizziness, palpitation, sallow face, pale tongue, thin pulse	Insufficiency of blood leading to poor source of menstruation	Blood deficiency

Scant menstruation, purple-colored vaginal blood with clots, abdominal pain, purple tongue, choppy pulse	Qi stagnation or cold restricting the circulation of the blood and blocking the chong and ren channels	Blood stasis

3. IRREGULAR MENSTRUAL CYCLE

An irregular menstrual cycle is one characterized by an inconsistent number of days between the onsets of successive periods (see Table 4.62).

Table 4.62 Irregular Menstrual Cycle

Manifestations	Pathogenesis	Clinical Pattern
Irregular menstruation, dark and scant menstruation with pain in the hypochondrium and distension around the breasts	Emotional depression leading to qi stagnation	Qi stagnation
Irregular menstruation, light-colored and thin menstruation with soreness of the lumbar area and knees, lassitude and listlessness	Insufficiency of liver and kidney yin leading to poor nourishment of the chong and ren channels	Liver-kidney yin deficiency

4. METRORRHAGIA

Metrorrhagia refers to a condition characterized by irregular uterine bleeding between the menstruation periods (see Table 4.63).

4.63 Metrorrhagia

Manifestations	Pathogenesis	Clinical Pattern
Metrorrhagia, dark-colored and thick menstruation, thirst, irritability, constipation, red tongue, rapid pulse	Heat accumulating in the body and forcing blood out of the vessels	Excess heat
Metrorrhagia, light-colored and thin menstruation, pale face, poor appetite, loose stools, leucorrhea, weak pulse	Insufficiency of spleen and kidney qi leading to poor consolidation of the chong and ren channels	Spleen-kidney qi deficiency
Metrorrhagia, dark thick menstruation with blood clots, abdominal pain, purple tongue with ecchymosis and petechia, choppy pulse	Blood stagnating in the chong and ren channels	Blood stasis

5. AMENORRHEA

Amenorrhea presents as two different conditions. One refers to the absence of menarche in a female over 18 years old; the other refers to the absence of menstruation for over three successive months in a female who has already begun to menstruate. Amenorrhea can be identified as different patterns depending on the causes (see Table 4.64).

Table 4.64 Amenorrhea

Manifestations	Pathogenesis	Clinical Pattern
Amenorrhea with pale face, lips, and nails, dizziness, blurred vision with floaters, thin pulse	Insufficiency of blood leading to poor nourishment of chong and ren channels	Blood deficiency
Amenorrhea with abdominal pain or hard masses, purple tongue, choppy pulse; occurring in cases of uterine fibroids, ovarian cysts, and cancers of the reproductive system	Blockage of blood vessels leading to stagnation of the flow of blood	Blood stasis
Amenorrhea, abdominal pain with cold sensation relieved by warmth, pale tongue, deep slow pulse	Cold accumulating in the chong and ren channels	Excess cold

6. DYSMENORRHEA

Dysmenorrhea refers to abdominal pain related to the menstrual cycle. Dysmenorrhea is clinically identified as several pattern types as shown in Table 4.65.

Table 4.65 Dysmenorrhea

Manifestations	Pathogenesis	Clinical Pattern
Dysmenorrhea occurring **before or during** menstruation, with distending or stabbing pain in the lower abdomen before menstruation	Qi stagnation and blood stasis leading to obstruction of the uterine network vessels	Qi-blood stagnation
Dysmenorrhea marked by a vague hollow pain in the lower abdomen **after** menstruation, pale face, soreness and weakness of the lumbar area and knees, weak pulse	Insufficiency of blood leading to poor nourishment of the chong and ren channels	Blood deficiency

Dysmenorrhea occurring during menstruation with a history of cold attack, marked by severe pain with cold sensation of the lower abdomen relieved by warmth	Cold accumulating in the chong and ren channels	Excess cold

XI. ABNORMAL LEUCORRHEA

Abnormal leucorrhea includes excessive leucorrhea or dribbling leucorrhea with changes in color, thickness, and odor.

Key Signs for Interrogation

Color, amount, thickness, and odor (see Table 4.66).

Table 4.66 Abnormal Leucorrhea

Manifestations	Pathogenesis	Clinical Pattern
Profuse, light-colored, and thin leucorrhea without foul odor, poor appetite, loss of taste, loose stools, lassitude, and weak pulse	Insufficiency of spleen-kidney yang leading to poor consolidation of the chong and ren channels	Spleen-kidney yang deficiency
Profuse thin, white vaginal discharge without odor, distending pain of the lower abdomen, poor appetite, nausea and vomiting, heavy sensation of the head and body, soft slow pulse	Cold damp accumulating in the spleen and stomach leading to vaginal discharge below	Cold damp
Profuse yellow and thick vaginal discharge with foul odor, abdominal pain, yellow greasy tongue coating, rolling rapid pulse	Damp heat accumulating in the liver and gallbladder leading to discharge below	Damp heat
Vaginal discharge with blood, abdominal pain; occurring in cases of pelvic infection or cervical cancer	Excess heat stagnating in the liver channel and impairing the uterine network vessels	Liver heat; damp heat
Persistent profuse bloody vaginal discharge after menopause, abdominal pain or hard masses, occurring in cases of cancer of the reproductive system	Qi and blood stagnation in the chong and ren channels	Qi-blood stagnation

XII. DISORDERS DURING PREGNANCY

In a normal physiological state, a woman might suffer from some mild symptoms during a pregnancy which do not require treatment. This section will discuss those manifestations that are intolerably severe or which are abnormal.

1. VOMITING

Normally vomiting may occur during pregnancy, but generally disappears within three months. If vomiting lasts more than three months, possibly becoming more severe, treatment is necessary (see Table 4.67).

Table 4.67 Vomiting

Manifestations	Pathogenesis	Clinical Pattern
Vomiting with lassitude and listlessness, loss of taste, and distension of the abdomen, loose stools, weak rolling pulse	Insufficiency of spleen qi leading to poor promotion of stomach qi	Spleen qi deficiency
Severe vomiting, with irritability, bitter taste in mouth and acid reflux, moodiness, wiry rolling pulse	Liver fire transversely attacking the stomach leading to reversal of stomach qi	Liver fire
Nausea and vomiting with fullness of the upper abdomen, poor appetite, heaviness of the body, edema, greasy tongue coating	Turbid phlegm accumulating in the stomach leading to reversal of stomach qi	Phlegm

2. THREATENED MISCARRIAGE

Threatened miscarriage not only refers to irregular vaginal bleeding during pregnancy but also to severe soreness of the lumbosacral area and abdominal pain with a downbearing sensation (see Table 4.68).

Table 4.68 Threatened Miscarriage

Manifestations	Pathogenesis	Clinical Pattern
Irregular vaginal bleeding, pale face, lips, and nails, lassitude, dizziness, pale tongue, weak rolling pulse	Insufficiency of both qi and blood resulting in poor nourishment of the fetus	Qi-blood deficiency
Bloody vaginal discharge with downbearing pain in the lower abdomen radiating to the lumbosacral area, dusky face with pigmented spots, dizziness and tinnitus, frequent urination	Insufficiency of kidney qi leading to lack of consolidation in the chong and ren channels	Kidney qi deficiency

	Trauma impairing fetal qi (which is rooted in kidney qi) leading to lack of consolidation of the fetus	Insecurity of kidney qi
Vaginal bleeding occurring after sprains, contusions, or other traumatic injuries		

3. Habitual Miscarriage

Habitual miscarriage refers to miscarriage occurring more than three times in succession (see Table 4.69).

Table 4.69 Habitual Miscarriage

Manifestations	Pathogenesis	Clinical Pattern
Miscarriage, facial palor, pale lips and nails, lassitude, dizziness, numbness or tingling of the fingers and toes, pale tender tongue, weak thin rolling pulse	Insufficiency of both qi and blood leading to poor nourishment and promotion in the chong and ren channels	Qi-blood deficiency
Miscarriage, downbearing pain in the lower abdomen radiating to the lumbosacral area, dusky face with pigmented spots, dizziness and tinnitus, frequent urination, lower back pain, weak knees	Insufficiency of kidney qi leading to poor consolidation in the chong and ren channels	Kidney qi deficiency

XIII. Postpartum Disorders

According to TCM, an impairment of qi and blood will occur after childbirth. Owing to a woman's weakened condition in this special period, the body is easily affected by pathogenic factors.

Key Signs for Interrogation

Color, amount, thickness, and odor of vaginal discharge, and fever.

1. Persistent Lochia

Normally, the lochia will disappear within a week after birth following the involution of the uterus. Persistent lochia of a normal or abnormal color or odor should be examined (see Table 4.70).

Table 4.70 Persistent Lochia

Manifestations	Pathogenesis	Clinical Pattern
Lingering vaginal bleeding of a light color following birth, with sallow face, listlessness and lassitude, vague pain in the lower abdomen, weak pulse	Insufficiency of spleen qi resulting in dysfunction in keeping the blood within the vessels	Spleen qi deficiency
Persistent thick bloody vaginal discharge of a dark color, with a foul odor, flushed face, thirst, constipation, fever, scant urine, rapid pulse	Heat in the blood level accumulating in the body and damaging the uterine network vessels	Blood heat
Persistent lochia containing blood clots, stabbing pain of the lower abdomen, purple tongue with ecchymosis and petechiae, choppy pulse	Stagnation of blood in the uterus	Blood stasis

2. POSTPARTUM FEVER

Fever occurring after birth is common with various puerperal infections (see Table 4.71).

Table 4.71 Postpartum Fever

Manifestations	Pathogenesis	Clinical Pattern
Fever, chills, headache, aching, lack of perspiration, and floating pulse	Invasion of wind cold leading to tightness of the muscular interstices	Exterior
High fever, irritability, yellow urine, constipation, red tongue, rapid pulse	Excess heat accumulating in the interior of the body	Excess heat
Low-grade fever with dizziness, vertigo, dry bowels, vague abdominal pain, pale tongue and nails, thin pulse	Insufficiency of blood causing internal dryness and deficiency heat	Blood deficiency

XIV. DISORDERS OF INFANTS

The normal physiological characteristics of an infant present as delicate and immature functioning of the internal organs, a rapid speed of development, and vigorous movements. Pathological characteristics in an infant appear as a sudden attack by pathogenic factors, a labile state during illness, or, most commonly, digestive and respiratory disorders.

1. Conditions Occurring Before or Soon after Birth

Disorders before or soon after birth refer to those occurring in infants from birth to three years old.

Disorders of the newborn (birth to three months) are mostly related to congenital factors or events occurring during delivery, including nutrition of the mother during pregnancy, premature labor, difficult labor, cesarean section, or forceps delivery.

Disorders of the infant from one to three years old are mainly related to feeding. Improper feeding may lead to five different kinds of flaccidity: flaccidity of the neck, upper back, extremities, muscles, and mastication; or to five different kinds of retardation: delayed development in standing, walking, hair growth, teething, and the faculty of speech. Improper feeding also causes infantile malnutrition.

2. Vaccination for the Prevention of Disease

Infants from six months to five years old have lost their congenital immunity, but their acquired immunity has not yet been built up. Thus, an infant is liable to contract infectious disorders during this period. The practitioner should inquire about the infant's history of vaccinations and contagious diseases, as well as determine whether the child has had contact with anyone suffering from a communicable disease.

3. Interrogation about Etiological Factors

Owing to the immature development of the nervous system, the infant is liable to be easily frightened and to suffer from high fever and convulsions. Due to an underdeveloped ability to digest food, an infant is also liable to suffer from indigestion which is manifested by vomiting, diarrhea, and malnutrition. Because of poor adaptability to the external environment, an infant is liable to be more easily affected by external pathogenic factors, commonly manifested in conditions such as fever, cough, or asthma.

CHAPTER FIVE

Pulse Examination and Palpation

Although pulse examination and palpation are considered a single activity, they consist of two distinct methods. Pulse examination is a special diagnostic skill of TCM and includes the location, frequency, rhythm, shape, and amplitude of the pulse. Palpation serves to find abnormal signs by touching, feeling, pressing, and tapping on the surface of the body.

I. PULSE EXAMINATION

Pulse examination is an important aspect of TCM, and is historically considered to be one of the most brilliant components of TCM diagnostic methods.

1. THE THEORY OF PULSE EXAMINATION ON CUN KOU

The textual source for the theory of feeling the pulse on *cun kou* can be found in the *Huang Di Nei Jing* (*Yellow Emperor's Classic of Internal Medicine*), which was written over 2000 years ago. It was described in detail in the *Nan Jing* (*Classic of Difficulties*), which was completed during the Han Dynasty, and it was adopted by the time of the *Mai Jing* (*Pulse Classic*). Cun kou refers to an area close to the wrist where the radial artery beats. There are many reasons for feeling the pulse on cun kou:

• Cun kou is located at the place where the lung channel of hand tai yin crosses over, and the lung channel originates from the middle burner that serves as the source of qi and blood.

• According to TCM theory, cun kou, at *Tai Yuan* (LU-9) is a place where the vessels meet, so it can show the changes of qi and blood in all vessels.

• The radial artery becomes anatomically more shallow around cun kou and there is adequate space for finger placement.

• Using the radial bone as a support, performing pulse examination on cun kou is both practical and convenient.

2. FORMATION OF PULSE

TCM teaches that the heart and the blood vessels are the main organ and tissues responsible for forming a pulse. Circulating inside the vessels, qi and blood are the basis of the pulse; the lung governs respiration and qi, which promotes, restores, and consolidates the circulation of blood; the spleen and stomach are responsible for transporting and transforming foodstuff and refined nutritious substances, which serve as the source of qi and blood; the liver stores blood and also disperses it by smoothing the flow of qi and blood in the vessels; the kidney stores essence, from which primordial qi is derived. In the light of TCM, primordial qi acts as the primary motive force for the circulation of blood and other life activities.

3. LOCATION AND METHODS FOR PULSE EXAMINATION

Cun Kou Pulse Examination

Cun kou pulse examination is a diagnostic method using the pulsation of the radial artery, which is located medial to the radial styloid process, to determine the healthy and pathological state of the patient.

There are three pulse positions at cun kou, namely *cun, guan*, and *chi*. The point which is level with the radial styloid process is guan; cun is located distal to guan (closer to the wrist); and chi is located proximal to guan (closer to the elbow). Within cun, guan, and chi, each position has three levels, namely superficial, middle, and deep; thus, in total, there are nine regions.

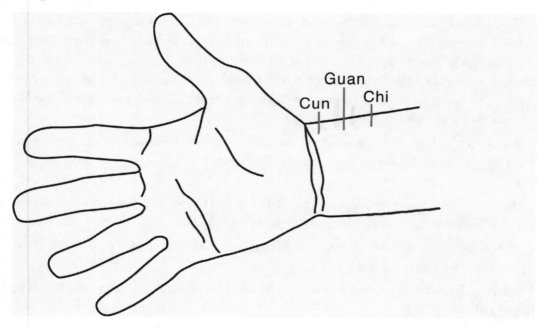

Figure 5.1: Pulse Location for Overall Cun Kou Pulse Reading

In TCM literature, there are different classifications for cun kou pulse examination, which are shown in Table 5.1.

Table 5.1 Relations between Positions and Internal Organs in Cun Kou

Text	Cun		Guan		Chi	
	Left	Right	Left	Right	Left	Right
Nan Jing (Difficult Classic)	HT	LU	LR	SP	KI	KI
	SI	LI	GB	ST	BL	Life Gate
Mai Jing (Pulse Classic)	HT	LU	LR	SP	KI	KI
	SI	LI	GB	ST	BL	TB
Jing Yue Quan Shu (Collected Treatises of Jing Yue)	HT	LU	LR	SP	KI	KI
	PC	*Tan Zhong* (CV-17)	GB	ST	BL, LI	TB, Life Gate, SI
Yi Jong Jin Jian (Golden Mirror of the Medical Tradition)	HT	LU	LR	SP	KI	KI
	Tan Zhong (CV-17)	Chest	Diaphragm, GB	ST	BL, SI	LI

Overall Pulse Examination

In a general sense, pulse examination refers to the diagnostic method which uses the arteries located at three different positions of the body, i.e., an upper position (head), middle position (hand) and lower position (foot). Each position has three areas, i.e. heaven, humankind, and earth. Altogether, there are nine regions (see Table 5.2 and Figure 5.2).

Table 5.2 General Pulse Examination and Clinical Significance

Three Positions	Nine Regions	Relevant Channel and Point	Relevant Artery	Relevant Area or Region
Upper (head)	Heaven	Foot shao yang, *Tai Yang* (extra point)	Temporal artery	Side of head

	Earth	Foot yang ming, *Ju Liao* (ST-3)	Facial artery	Teeth and mouth
	Humanity	Hand shao yang, *Er Men* (TB-21)	Temporal artery	Ears and eyes
Middle (hand)	Heaven	Hand tai yin, *Tai Yuan* (LU-9), *Jing Qu* (LU-8)	Radial artery	Lung
	Earth	Hand yang ming, *He Gu* (LI-4)	Radial artery	Chest
	Humanity	Hand shao yin, *Shen Men* (HT-7)	Ulnar artery	Heart
Lower (foot)	Heaven	Foot jue yin, *Tai Chong* (LR-3), *Wu Li* (LR-10)	Dorsal artery; Femoral artery	Liver
	Earth	Foot shao yin, *Tai Xi* (KI-3)	Tibial artery	Kidney
	Humanity	Foot tai yin, *Ji Men* (SP-11); Foot yang ming, *Chong Yang* (ST-42)	Femoral artery; Dorsal artery	Spleen, stomach

Fig 5.2 Pulse Positions of the Three Areas and Nine Regions

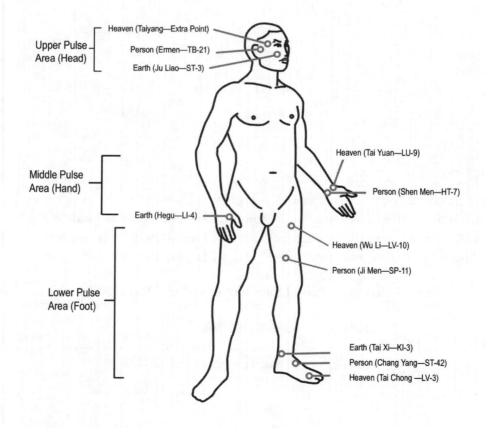

Diagnosis in Traditional Chinese Medicine

4. KEY POINTS TO NOTE

Environment

For pulse examination, the external environment must be quiet. The internal environment, referring to the practitioner, should be calm and concentrated, with uniform respiration. One reason for this is that the practitioner has to count pulse beats according to the respiratory cycle. Another reason is that peaceful respiration aids the practitioner in concentrating in order to carefully examine the condition of the pulse.

Positioning the Arm

The patient may sit or lie down. The patient should relax and naturally extend the forearm with the palm up and level with the heart. A small padded pulse pillow is placed under the wrist to clearly expose cun kou.

Placing the Fingers

The practitioner should keep the fingers on cun kou, the index finger at the cun position, the middle finger at guan, and the ring finger at chi. The tips of the three fingers should be arranged along a straight line (see Figure 5.1). It may be necessary to lift two of the three fingers slightly to feel carefully at the third position.

The fingers should be placed according to the patient's body type, i.e., more widely spaced for a taller patient, and closer together for a shorter person. Due to the shortness of cun kou in an infant, the practitioner often uses only one finger (thumb or index finger) to feel the pulse.

Finger Pressure

The practitioner feels the pulse by pushing the fingers back and forth in order to find the best position and amount of pressure for an accurate reading. There are three degrees of finger pressure for pulse examination.

- *Superficial level:* The practitioner exerts only slight pressure on the artery.
- *Middle level:* The practitioner feels the pulse by exerting more substantial pressure.
- *Deep level:* The practitioner presses the pulse down to the radial bone.

Duration

A pulse examination traditionally requires more than three minutes for each hand.

Factors to Take into Account

Seasons. A normal pulse is relatively wiry in spring, full in summer, superficial in fall, and deep in winter.

Sex. Women's pulses are naturally slightly softer and more rapid than men's. Also, the pulse is rolling, rapid, and peaceful during pregnancy.

Age. In general, the younger the person, the faster the pulse rate. Normal rates vary, but their ranges are shown in Table 5.3.

Table 5.3 Normal Variations of Heart Rate

Age (years)	Rate (beats/min)
0–1	120–140
1–4	90–110
4–10	80–90
10–16	76–80
16–35	70–76
35–50	70–72
50+	60–70

Normal Pulse Condition and Body Type

The pulse condition is closely related to the patients' body type (see Table 5.4).

Table 5.4 Normal Pulse Condition and Body Type

Pulse Condition	Body type
Longer	Tall
Shorter	Short
Deeper	Obese
More superficial	Slender

Occupation

The pulse is stronger in people who are engaged in heavy physical labor than in those engaged in mental work. Other factors may also influence the pulse condition, including medications, exercise, emotional factors, and food intake.

5. EIGHT QUALITIES OF A PULSE

There are eight different qualities that are taken into consideration when describing a pulse. These are shown in Table 5.5.

Table 5.5 Eight Qualities of a Pulse

Qualities	Indication	Examples
Location	Depth of pulse	*Floating pulse*: located superficially *Deep pulse*: located deeper

Frequency	Beats per respiratory cycle	*Rapid pulse*: 6 beats per cycle *Slow pulse*: 3 beats per cycle
Length	Scale of pulse in length	*Long pulse*: longer than *cun*, *guan*, and *chi* together *Short pulse*: shorter than the three positions
Strength	Force of pulse against the belly of the fingers	*Replete pulse*: forceful beating *Weak pulse*: forceless beating
Width	Scale of pulse in width	*Flooding pulse*: wider than normal *Thin pulse*: thinner than normal, even thread-like
Smoothness	Fluidity of pulse	*Rolling pulse*: smooth and rounded *Choppy pulse*: rough and hard-driving
Tension	Tightness of pulse	*Wiry pulse*: straight and tense like a guitar string *Moderate pulse*: gentle and loose
Rhythm	Uniformity in rhythm of beat and strength against the fingers	*Knotted pulse*: slow pulse with irregular missing beats *Hurried pulse*: rapid pulse with irregular missing beats *Intermittent pulse*: pulse with regular missing beats

6. GENERAL CLINICAL SIGNIFICANCE

Pulse examination can significantly reflect different aspects of an illness (see Table 5.6) including location, property, constitutional situation, and prognosis.

Table 5.6 General Clinical Significance of the Pulse Condition

Clinical Significance	Example	
	Pulse condition	**Pattern indication**
Determine location of an illness	Floating pulse	Exterior
	Deep pulse	Interior
Determine properties of an illness	Slow pulse	Cold
	Rapid pulse	Heat
Determine weakness or prevalence of vital qi and pathogenic factors	Weak pulse	Qi deficiency
	Flooding pulse	Excess heat

| Determine prognosis of an illness | Pulse with moderate location, speed, strength, rhythm, and tension | Existence of stomach qi and a good prognosis |
| | Roof-leaking pulse (see Table 5.16) | Exhaustion of stomach qi and a poor prognosis |

7. NORMAL PULSE CONDITION

There are three groups of manifestations for a normal pulse that can determine the presence of stomach qi, vitality, and root. (A pulse characterized as having a root refers to a condition in which pulsation can still be felt when forcefully pressing at the chi position.) These manifestations are shown in Table 5.7.

Table 5.7 Normal Pulse Condition

Determination	Manifestations
Presence of stomach qi *(wèi qì)*	Moderate in location, speed, strength, rhythm, and tension
Presence of vitality *(shén)*	Pulse is gentle and forceful under the fingers
Presence of root *(gēn)*	Pulse can be felt when forcefully pressing at chi position

8. ABNORMAL PULSE CONDITIONS

In TCM literature, the classifications and nomenclature for pulse conditions are often quite diverse, but almost all pulse conditions are categorized according to the location, frequency, and other qualities. This section includes twenty-seven kinds of commonly seen pulses according to eight qualities. In addition, the seven true visceral pulse conditions will be examined.

Key Signs for Pulse Examination

Look for pulses with any of the following conditions out of norm: location, abnormal frequency, width, length, strength, smoothness, tension, and rhythm.

Pulses in Abnormal Locations

Pulses in abnormal locations refer to an abnormal depth of the pulse (see Table 5.8).

Table 5.8 Pulses in Abnormal Locations

Pulse	Description	Pathogenesis	Clinical Pattern
Floating pulse	Can be felt with light pressure of the fingers, just resting the fingers on the artery	Vital qi fighting with pathogens on exterior of the body	Exterior
		Declining yang qi flowing outwards	Yang exhaustion

Scattered pulse	Large, floating, and arrhythmic with uneven strength, disappears when pressed lightly	Unsteadiness of collapsed vital qi occurring in severe cases	Exhaustion
Hollow pulse	Floating, large, and hollow in the middle, as though the fingers were pressing on a scallion stalk	Right after bleeding or sudden body fluid loss such as severe vomiting or diarrhea, leading to sudden vital qi consumption in an excess constitution	Bleeding, body fluid collapse
Deep pulse	Can only be felt with heavy pressure of the fingers on the artery	Dysfunction of internal organs	Interior
Deep-seated pulse	Located deeper than deep pulse, felt only when the fingers press down to the radial bone	Loss of consciousness caused by conditions such as severe bacterial infection, loss of blood, sudden emotional stimulation, extreme pain	Reversal

Pulses with Abnormal Frequencies

Pulses with abnormal frequencies are characterized by an abnormal number of beats per respiratory cycle (see Table 5.9).

Table 5.9 Pulses with Abnormal Frequencies

Pulse	Manifestations	Clinical Pattern
Slow pulse	3 beats per respiratory cycle (under 60 beats per minute)	Excess cold pattern if forceful Deficiency cold pattern if forceless
Moderate pulse	4 beats per respiratory cycle (60-70 beats per minute)	Normal for healthy people Damp pattern
Rapid pulse	5-6 beats per respiratory cycle (over 90 beats per minute)	Excess heat pattern if forceful Deficiency heat pattern if forceless
Swift pulse	More than 7 beats per respiratory cycle (around 120 beats per minute)	Collapse of yin if forceful Collapse of yang if forceless

Pulses with Abnormal Width

Pulses with abnormal width can be either too wide or too narrow (see Table 5.10).

Table 5.10 Pulses with Abnormal Width

Pulse	Manifestations	Clinical Pattern
Flooding pulse	Feels large and long like surging waves when resting the fingers, full and forcefully bouncing up against the belly of the fingers, arriving vigorously and disappearing gently	Excess heat if forceful and rapid; yang deficiency if forceless and slow
Thin pulse	Feels thin and clear like a thread	Damp; qi-blood deficiency

Pulses with Abnormal Length

Pulses with abnormal length can be either too long or too short (see Table 5.11).

Table 5.11 Pulses with Abnormal Length

Pulse	Manifestations	Clinical significance
Long pulse	Longer than normal, extends slightly beyond the length of cun, guan, and chi	Yang; excess; heat
Short pulse	Occupies a shorter length than normal, only present at cun or guan, cannot be felt at the chi position	Qi stagnation if forceful Qi deficiency if forceless

Pulses with Abnormal Strength

Pulses with abnormal strength are those with abnormal force against the pads of the fingers (see Table 5.12).

Table 5.12 Pulses with Abnormal Strength

Pulse	Manifestations	Clinical Pattern
Weak pulse	Feels very soft and thin at the three positions and nine regions, disappears when stronger pressure is exerted	Qi deficiency; blood deficiency ; yin deficiency; yang deficiency
Feeble pulse	Extremely soft, thin, and deep and can only be felt when pressing deeply	Qi-blood deficiency; yang deficiency
Indistinct pulse	Feels extremely thin and soft, unclear underneath the fingers	Yang exhaustion; qi exhaustion

Pulses with Abnormal Smoothness

Pulses with abnormal smoothness are those without normal fluidity (see Table 5.13).

Table 5.13 Pulses with Abnormal Smoothness

Pulse	Manifestations	Clinical Pattern
Choppy pulse	Feels rough instead of smooth, like scraping a bamboo strip with a dull knife	Blood stasis; body fluids deficiency; blood deficiency
Rolling pulse	Feels smooth, rounded, slick to the fingers like beads rolling on a plate	Good health, particularly in young men if rolling and peaceful; women in pregnancy; excess heat; phlegm; food stagnation
Moving pulse	Feels rounded, rapid, and short like a bouncing bean, without definite shape, having no head or tail, just a rise in the center	Extreme pain; qi stagnation and blood stasis

Pulses with Abnormal Tension

Pulses with abnormal tension are those with abnormal tightness (see Table 5.14).

Table 5.14 Pulses with Abnormal Tension

Pulse	Manifestations	Clinical Significance
Wiry pulse	Feels taut and straight like pressing on a guitar string	Liver disorder; gallbladder impediment; phlegm; phlegm fluids
Tense pulse	Feels twisted like a thick rope, tighter and more forceful than wiry pulse	Excess cold; impediment pattern; stagnation of food
Tympanic pulse	Feels floating, hard, and tight at the superficial level and stretched like a drum	Bleeding, difficult labor, metrorrhagia, and impairment of kidney essence
Firm pulse	Can only be felt at the deep level and feels large, wiry, and long	Excess cold; qi stagnation and blood stasis
Soft pulse	Floating, thin, and soft	Qi and blood deficiency; damp

Pulses with Abnormal Rhythm

Pulses with abnormal rhythm are those without a regular beat (see Table 5.15).

Table 5.15 Pulses with Abnormal Rhythm

Pulse	Manifestations	Clinical Pattern
Knotted pulse	Feels slow and stops at irregular intervals	Stagnation of qi, blood, phlegm, cold, or food if forceful; deficiency of heart qi or heart blood
Hurried pulse	Feels hurried with irregular intervals	Collapse of vital qi or exhaustion of yin fluids if forceless; excess heat or stagnation of qi, blood, phlegm, or food if forceful
Intermittent pulse	Feels slow with regular intervals	Collapse of heart qi or blood if forceless; emotional distress if forceful; painful obstruction and severe traumatic injury

9. SEVEN TRUE VISCERAL PULSE CONDITIONS

These seven pulses are commonly found in those who are critically ill or dying (see Table 5.16).

Table 5.16 Seven True Visceral Pulse Conditions

Pulse	Manifestations	Clinical Pattern
Flicking-stone pulse	Pulse feels deep and solid, yet forceful, resembling flicking a stone with the finger tip	Evil qi attacking vital qi leading to collapse of stomach qi
Bubble-rising pulse	Floating like a bubble rising to the surface of boiling water	Extreme heat accumulating in three yang channels leading to exhaustion of body fluids
Fish-swimming pulse	Indistinct with intervals like a swimming fish intermittently floating up	Extreme cold accumulating in three yin channels leading to collapsed yang qi floating outwards
Shrimp-darting pulse	Nearly imperceptible pulse with occasional darting beats which resemble shrimp darting in water	Extreme cold accumulating in three yin channels leading to collapsed yang qi floating outwards

Diagnosis in Traditional Chinese Medicine

Roof-leaking pulse	Less than 40 beats per minute with irregular intervals like a roof leaking in the rain	Stomach qi exhaustion
Bird-pecking pulse	Pulse with rapid, irregular rhythm and intervals like a bird pecking food	Spleen qi exhaustion
Rope-untying pulse	At irregular intervals and arrhythmic, resembling the untying of a rope	Kidney qi exhaustion and collapse of life gate fire

10. COMPLEX PULSE CONDITIONS

In complex diseases, the pulse type usually presents as a combined form. Some common combinations are listed in Table 5.17.

Table 5.17 Combined Pulses Commonly Seen in Complex Diseases

Pulse	Clinical Significance
Floating tense pulse	Exterior cold; wind impediment
Floating moderate pulse	Exterior deficiency
Floating rapid pulse	Exterior heat
Floating rolling pulse	Wind phlegm; phlegm pattern combined with invasion of external pathogens
Deep slow pulse	Deficiency cold; excess cold
Wiry rapid pulse	Liver fire; liver qi stagnation; liver and gallbladder damp heat
Rolling rapid pulse	Phlegm heat; phlegm fire; excess heat; food stagnation
Flooding rapid pulse	Excess heat; qi level; yang ming bowel
Deep wiry pulse	Liver qi stagnation; body fluids retention
Deep choppy pulse	Blood stasis; excess cold
Wiry thin pulse	Liver yin-kidney yin deficiency; blood deficiency combined with liver qi stagnation; spleen deficiency combined with liver qi stagnation
Deep moderate pulse	Spleen deficiency–damp accumulation
Deep thin pulse	Yin deficiency; blood deficiency
Wiry rolling rapid pulse	Liver fire combined with phlegm; liver wind combined with phlegm fire

11. PULSES IN INFANTS

Owing to the shortened pulse location, a single finger is usually used for pulse examination in infants. The classification of pulses in infants is also simpler than that in adults. These pulses are shown in Table 5.18.

Table 5.18 Pulses in Infants

Pulse	Clinical Significance
Floating rapid pulse	Yang
Deep slow pulse	Yin
Floating rolling pulse	Wind
Deep rolling pulse	Food stagnation; phlegm
Rapid pulse	Heat
Slow pulse	Cold
Moderate pulse	Damp
Tense pulse	Impediment; cold

II. PALPATION

To judge the location, properties, and seriousness of a disorder, the practitioner may investigate the temperature, moisture, tension, swelling, presence of subcutaneous nodules, and tenderness, by touching, feeling, pressing, and tapping in certain areas of a patient's body. Palpation is an important part of the four diagnostic methods.

1. METHODS AND KEY POINTS TO NOTE

Using the correct methods for palpation enables the practitioner to obtain significant clinical information.

Methods for Palpation

There are four basic methods for palpation, including touching, feeling, pressing, and tapping.

Touching: The practitioner touches the forehead, extremities, or chest and abdomen of the patient with the fingers or the palm. The temperature and moisture of the skin can be examined by touching in order to identify exterior or interior patterns, the presence or absence of sweating, and the insufficiency or prevalence of yang qi and yin fluids.

Feeling: The practitioner feels the affected region with slight pressure. Feeling is used for the chest, abdomen, acupoints, or swollen areas. Local abnormal sensations such as pain or soreness, as well as the shape and size of a lump, can be known by feeling. This can be used to identify exterior or interior patterns, as well as deficiency or excess patterns.

Pressing: The practitioner applies deep pressure or pushes on a local area such as the chest or abdomen, or in a spot where a lump is located. Tenderness in a deeper part of the body, or the shape, hardness, properties, or mobility of a lump can be learned. This is used to identify deficiency or excess patterns and the weakness or strength of pathogens.

Tapping: The practitioner taps a certain area of the patient to induce a percussive sound and a vibration. This method is used to detect qi stagnation or retention of body fluids, along with the location and degree of an illness.

Points to Note

Sequence: Pressing should be done after touching and feeling. Tapping is done at the end. All four methods should begin lightly on the surface of the body and go from distal to proximal, and then applying increasing strength to reach the deeper parts of the body.

Precautions: Manipulations should be done gently and uniformly to avoid damage to the skin. Before palpation, the practitioner should warm his/her hands so the patient will be more comfortable.

Good cooperation: The practitioner should try to gain the confidence of the patient by observing the patient's changes of expression and inquiring frequently about the patient's well-being during palpitation.

2. CONTENTS OF PALPATION

Palpation is widely used in the clinic to examine the entire body. In TCM, there are certain points for attention in palpation that are similar to those in Western medicine, while some aspects are different. The latter are shown in the tables below.

Palpation of the Skin

Palpation of the skin is shown in Table 5.19.

Table 5.19 Palpation of the Skin

Manifestations	Pathogenesis	Clinical Pattern
The skin feels hot when initially touched, but becomes cooler if the touch is held longer	External heat stagnating on the surface of the body	Exterior heat
Feeling of heat increases with the length of the touch	Heat accumulating in the interior of the body	Interior heat

Manifestations	Pathogenesis	Clinical Pattern
Flaccid skin and muscles with preference for warmth and pressure	Insufficiency of yang qi leading to poor warmth and promotion of the body	Deficiency
Tight skin and muscles, tenderness	Pathogenic factors accumulating in the body	Excess
Pain occurring when just resting the fingers or palm on skin	Pathogens invading and staying on the surface of the body	Exterior
Pain felt only under forceful pressure	Pathogens entering and residing in the depths of the body	Interior
Dry and smooth skin	Absence of sweat without impairment of body fluids	Yin deficiency
Moist skin	Damp restricted inside the skin with poor distribution of yang qi	Yang deficiency
Scaly and dry skin	Blood stasis or severe impairment of yin fluids leading to poor nourishment of the skin	Blood stasis; yin deficiency
Indentation of the skin when pressing but returning to normal following the release of pressure	Qi stagnating in localized area	Qi stagnation
Indentation of the skin when pressing	Body fluids retained in the interior of the body	Damp; phlegm fluid
Redness, swelling, hot sensation, and pain	Heat accumulating in the skin	Excess heat
Swelling, hard masses with cold sensation	Cold accumulating in the skin	Excess cold

Palpation of the Limbs

Palpation of the limbs is shown in Table 5.20.

Table 5.20 Palpation of the Limbs

Manifestations	Pathogenesis	Clinical Pattern
Cold limbs occurring in acute or severe cases	Excess heat accumulating in the body and blocking yang qi from circulating outwards	Heat with false cold presentation

Cold limbs occurring in chronic cases	Insufficiency of yang qi leading to poor warmth of the limbs	Deficiency cold
Coldness in all fingertips in infants; symptomatic of impending infantile convulsion	Excess heat stirring up liver wind	Liver wind
Coldness of the middle fingertip, symptomatic of impending measles or chickenpox	Toxic heat accumulating internally and blocking yang qi from circulating outwards	Toxic heat
Hot limbs	Excess heat steaming outward	Excess heat
Five-palm heat	Insufficiency of yin fluids producing deficiency heat	Deficiency heat
Hotness when touching both palms and soles	Steaming outward of external heat	Exterior heat

Palpation of the Neck

Palpation of the neck is shown in Table 5.21

Table 5.21 Palpation of the Neck

Manifestations	Pathogenesis	Clinical Pattern
Enlargement of thyroid gland with normal skin color, gland feels soft when palpated, as found in simple enlarged thyroid gland	Stagnated qi accumulating in the neck	Qi stagnation
One or several lumps which can be moved by pushing, no skin color change; occurring in thyroid fibroids	Qi stagnation accompanied by accumulation of phlegm	Qi stagnation-phlegm accumulation
Enlargement of thyroid gland with uneven surface which feels hard and cannot be moved when pushed by the finger; occurring in thyroid cancer	Qi stagnation accompanied by blood stasis	Qi-blood stagnation
Inflamed lymph node or metastasis of cancer marked by single enlarged lymph node or plum pit	Qi stagnation accompanied by accumulation of phlegm	Qi stagnation-phlegm accumulation
Tuberculosis of lymph nodes with low-grade fever, night sweats, and five palm heat	Insufficiency of lung and kidney yin leading to production of deficiency fire	Lung yin-kidney yin deficiency

Palpation of the Chest and Hypochondrium

Palpation of the chest and hypochondrium is shown in Table 5.22.

Table 5.22 Palpation of the Chest and Hypochondrium

Manifestations	Clinical Pattern
Diminution of heartbeat	Ancestral qi deficiency
Intensification of heartbeat	Outgoing of ancestral qi
Powerful heartbeat with poor health condition, or no heartbeat	Collapse of heart qi
Powerful heartbeat before or after birth labor	Severe condition
Stuffy thoracic region, oppression of the chest	Qi stagnation
Distending pain with pressure	Accumulation of phlegm heat accompanied by qi stagnation or phlegm fluids retention

Palpation of the Abdomen

Palpation of the abdomen is shown in Table 5.23.

Table 5.23 Palpation of the Abdomen

Manifestations	Pathogenesis	Clinical Pattern
Cold sensation when touching abdominal region, abdominal pain relieved by pressing and warmth	Deficiency of yang qi leading to poor warmth	Deficiency cold
Hot sensation when touching abdominal region, preference for cold, tenderness	Excess heat stirring up inside the body	Excess heat
Vague pain of the abdomen, preference for pressure	Insufficiency of yang qi leading to poor warmth and promotion of qi and blood	Deficiency
Severe pain of abdomen, tenderness aggravated by pressure	Qi or food stagnation leading to blood stasis, or accumulation of parasites in intestines	Excess

Distension and fullness of the abdomen, tenderness	Accumulation of dry stools, stagnation of undigested food, or retention of body fluids	Excess
Abdominal distension without tenderness, tympany when knocked	Qi stagnation occurring in intestines without presence of material pathogens	Qi stagnation
Distension and fullness of the chest and gastric region with pain when pushing down, cough with sticky sputum	Accumulation of phlegm heat in the chest obstructing the flow of qi	Phlegm heat
Fullness in the epigastrium, flaccid skin and muscles when pushing down	Qi stagnation occurring in upper abdomen	Qi stagnation
Severe pain of the lower abdomen aggravated by pressure, tenderness and even fever	Accumulation of toxic heat in the intestines	Excess heat
Abdominal masses which can be dispersed by pressure, migrating pain	Invisible qi stagnating in the abdomen, moving from one area to another	Qi stagnation
Abdominal masses which can not be dispersed by pressure, stabbing pain fixed at a certain area	Congealed blood stagnating in the abdomen, and fixed in a certain area	Blood stasis

Palpation on the Acupoints

Acupuncture points are physiologically and pathologically related to the function of *zang* or *fu* organs via the channels and network vessels with the same name as the organ. So an abnormal manifestation at an acupoint can be used to detect disorders of the internal organs.

Common abnormal manifestations at these points are tenderness, hypersensitivity, or cord-shaped lumps or nodes (see Table 5.24).

Table 5.24 Palpation of the Points

Location of Disorder	Manifestations	Point
Lung	Tenderness, hard lumps	*Fei Shu* (BL 13), *Tai Yuan* (LU-9), *Zhong Fu* (LU-1)
Heart	Tenderness, soreness	*Ju Que* (CV-14), *Tan Zhong* (CV-17), *Da Ling* (PC-7)

Liver	Tenderness, soreness	*Gan Shu* (BL 18), *Tai Chong* (LR-3), *Qi Men* (LR-14)
Spleen	Tenderness, soreness	*Zhang Men* (LR-13), *Tai Bai* (SP-3), *Pi Shu* (BL-20)
Kidney	Tenderness, soreness	*Qi Hai* (CV-6), *Tai Xi* (KI-3), *Shen Shu* (BL-23)
Large Intestine	Tenderness	*Tian Shu* (ST-25), *Da Chang Shu* (BL-25)
Small Intestine	Tenderness	*Guan Yuan* (CV-4), *Xiao Chang Shu* (BL-27)
Gallbladder	Tenderness	*Ri Yue* (GB-24), *Dan Shu* (BL-19)
Stomach	Tenderness	*Wei Shu* (BL-21), *Zu San Li* (ST-36)
Bladder	Tenderness	*Zhong Ji* (CV-3), *Ci Liao* (BL-32)

PART TWO

Pattern Identification

Pattern Identification According to the Eight Principles

Pattern identification according to the eight principles should be the first step in classifying the complex manifestations learned from the four diagnostic methods. The eight principles refer to eight categories according to which patterns are named and differentiated. These are exterior, interior, cold, heat, deficiency, excess, yin, or yang.

I. A GENERAL UNDERSTANDING OF THE EIGHT PRINCIPLES

Before covering pattern identification, a general understanding of each of the eight principles is necessary. The tables below show the basic pathogenesis and clinical significance of the eight principles by grouping them into opposing pairs.

1. EXTERIOR AND INTERIOR

Exterior and interior comprise the pair of principles that indicate the location of a disorder (see Table 6.1).

Table 6.1 Exterior and Interior

Principle	Pathogenesis	Clinical Pattern
Exterior	External pathogenic factors attacking the exterior of the body—the skin, hair follicles, muscular interstices, channels, and network vessels level	Exterior
Interior	Pathogenic factors impairing the internal organs, qi and blood; or dysfunction of the internal organs, qi and blood–the organs, bone, marrow, qi, and blood level	Interior

2. COLD AND HEAT

Cold and heat comprise the pair of principles that indicate the property/nature of a disorder (see Table 6.2).

Table 6.2 Cold and Heat

Principle	Pathogenesis	Clinical Pattern
Cold	Cold attacking the body; or insufficiency of yang qi producing internal cold	Cold
Heat	Heat attacking the body, or insufficiency of yin fluids producing internal heat	Heat

3. DEFICIENCY AND EXCESS

Deficiency and excess are the pair of principles that indicate the weakness or prevalence of vital qi versus pathogenic factors (see Table 6.3).

Table 6.3 Deficiency and Excess

Principle	Pathogenesis	Clinical Pattern
Deficiency	Weakness of vital qi	Deficiency
Excess	Prevalence of pathogenic factors with strong vital qi	Excess

4. YIN AND YANG

Yin and yang comprise the pair of principles that indicate the classification of a disorder. Generally speaking, yin comprises interior, cold, and deficiency patterns, while yang comprises exterior, heat, and excess patterns. Yin and yang are the most basic of the eight principles (see Table 6.4).

Table 6.4 Yin and Yang

Principle	Pathogenesis	Clinical Pattern
Yin	Pathogens as well as the illness itself presenting yin properties	Interior; cold; deficiency
Yang	Pathogens as well as the illness itself presenting yang properties	Exterior; heat; excess

According to TCM theory, yin and yang have particular and specific meanings in clinical practice. Basic patterns of yin and yang imbalance include yin deficiency or excess, and yang deficiency or excess. These will be discussed under the eight principles below. As two extreme conditions in the clinic, yin and yang exhaustion patterns will also be reviewed under the eight principles.

Yin and yang in relation to each individual organ (such as heart yang, heart yin, stomach yang, stomach yin, kidney yang, and kidney yin) will be discussed in Chapter Nine, "Pattern Identification According to the Internal Organs."

II. Patterns According to the Eight Principles

Pattern identification according to the eight principles means applying the theory of the eight principles in order to analyze a patient's general condition and then identify the location and properties of a disorder, the condition of vital qi and pathogens, and the classification of patterns.

This method is the most important type of pattern identification and the first step of diagnosis. It will classify all the manifestations collected by the four diagnostic methods under individual principles (such as deficiency or heat) and/or their combinations (such as excess heat, exterior cold). The patterns identified by this method are only preliminary diagnoses.

The manifestations will then be analyzed macroscopically based on the practitioner's understanding of the state of qi, blood, and the internal organs. The preliminary diagnosis gained on the basis of the eight principles will be further classified on the basis of the condition of qi, blood, and the internal organs to achieve the final pattern. The final pattern refers to the one on which treatment principle and treatment should be based.

1. Exterior Patterns

This refers to the group of patterns that occur on the exterior of the body; they are caused by an invasion of the body's exterior by external pathogens. The diagnosis of an exterior pattern is therefore clinically determined by two conditions:

- The location of an exterior pattern must be the exterior of the body.
- The pathogens that cause an exterior pattern must be external pathogens.

Depending on the invading external pathogens and the corresponding reactions of the body, exterior patterns can be further classified into exterior cold patterns or exterior heat patterns. The former includes both exterior excess patterns and exterior deficiency patterns.

General Overview

An overview of exterior patterns is shown in Table 6.5.

Table 6.5 General Overview of Exterior Patterns

Main Diagnostic Points	Common Pathogenesis	Common Patterns
Disorders occurring in the exterior of the body; shorter illness process; mild severity of illness presentation; at the early stage of a disorder	External pathogenic factors attacking the exterior of the body	Exterior cold (including exterior deficiency and exterior excess pattern); exterior heat

Common pathogenesis

Exterior patterns can be further differentiated as cold or heat, both of which are combined with wind manifestations and are related to different pathogeneses. The manifestations and analyses of each pathogenesis are shown in Tables 6.6 and 6.7.

Table 6.6 Exterior Cold Patterns

Common Pathogenesis	
External pathogenic wind cold attacking the exterior of the body	
Manifestations	**Systematic Pathogenesis**
Chills greater than fever, or aversion to wind	Dysfunction of wei qi in dispersing
Headaches, soreness and discomfort of the whole body	Obstruction of qi in the channels and network vessels
Stuffiness of nose, runny nose, sneezing, and slight cough	Dysfunction of the lung in dispersing and precipitating qi
Thin white tongue coating and floating tense/moderate pulse	Pathogenic cold remaining in the exterior of the body

Table 6.7 Exterior Heat Patterns

Common Pathogenesis	
External pathogenic wind heat attacking the exterior of the body	
Manifestations	**Systematic Pathogenesis**
Fever greater than chills, or aversion to cold	Dysfunction of wei qi in dispersing
Headaches, soreness and discomfort of the whole body	Obstruction of qi in the channels and network vessels
Runny nose with yellow nasal discharge, cough, sore throat, and slight thirst	Dysfunction of the lung in dispersing and precipitating qi
Thin yellow tongue coating and floating rapid pulse	Pathogenic heat remaining in the exterior of the body

2. INTERIOR PATTERNS

This refers to patterns that are located in the depths of the body and involve qi, blood, and the internal organs.

General overview

A general overview of interior patterns is shown in Table 6.8.

Table 6.8 General Overview of Interior Patterns

Main Diagnostic Points	Pathogenesis	Common Patterns
Disorders occurring in the interior of the body; lingering illness process; more serious degree of illness presentation; occurring at the late stage of a disorder	External pathogenic factors entering and accumulating in the internal organs, qi, and blood; or dysfunction of the internal organs, qi, and blood	Excess heat; deficiency heat; deficiency cold; excess cold

Common Manifestations

Interior patterns include those with deficiency and excess, as well as those with heat and cold manifestations. The pathogeneses are different for each combination. In clinical practice, interior patterns are mainly classified as excess heat patterns, excess cold patterns, deficiency heat patterns, and deficiency cold patterns. Of the latter two patterns, deficiency heat patterns are also referred to as yin deficiency patterns because yin deficiency leads to the production of internal heat. Deficiency cold patterns are also called yang deficiency patterns because yang deficiency results in the generation of internal cold.

The common manifestations and analyses of each pathogenesis are shown in Tables 6.9 to 6.12.

Table 6.9 Manifestations and Pathogenesis of Excess Heat Patterns

Common Pathogenesis	
Excess heat accumulating in the interior of the body	
Manifestations	**Systematic Pathogenesis**
Fever, malar flush, and sensation of heat in the limbs	Excess heat dispersing outward
Profuse sweating	Excess heat steaming body fluids outward
Thirst with desire to drink	Excess heat impairing yin fluids

Dry stools	Poor moistening of the intestinal tract
Scant urine	Impairment of body fluids leading to a poor source of urine
Irritability and possibly delirium	Upward flaring of excess heat affecting the mind
Red tongue with yellow dry coating; rolling, flooding, and rapid pulse	Accumulation of excess heat in the body

Table 6.10 Manifestations and Pathogenesis of Deficiency Heat/Yin Deficiency Patterns

Common Pathogenesis	
Insufficiency of yin fluids	
Manifestations	**Systematic Pathogenesis**
Tidal, hectic, or low-grade fever aggravated in the afternoon; night sweats	Deficiency heat retained inside the body and steaming yin fluids in the afternoon
Flushed zygomatic region	Rising of deficiency fire
Thirst without desire to drink	Poor moistening of the mouth
Dry stools	Poor lubrication of the intestinal tract
Scant dark colored urine	Impairment of body fluids
Irritability, five-palm heat	Stirring of deficiency fire inside the body
Red tongue with scant coating, thin and rapid pulse	Deficiency heat accumulating in the body

Table 6.11 Manifestations and Pathogenesis of Deficiency Cold/Yang Deficiency Patterns

Common Pathogenesis	
Insufficiency of yang qi	
Manifestations	**Systematic Pathogenesis**
Aversion to cold, cold limbs	Poor warmth of the whole body
Pale puffy face, pale and puffy tongue	Poor promotion of blood circulation or dysfunction in removing damp
Spontaneous sweating	Poor consolidation of the muscular interstices

Lack of thirst	Excess cold accumulating in the body
Loose stools	Dysfunction of transportation and transformation
Clear and excessive urine	Decline of life gate fire leading to poor consolidation of the bladder
Distinctive or deep and slow pulse with forceless beating	Poor promotion of the blood vessels
Pain in the abdomen, preference for warmth and pressure	Warmth restores yang, while pressure reinforces excess

Table 6.12 Manifestations and Pathogenesis of Excess Cold Patterns

Common Pathogenesis	
Excess cold accumulating in the interior of the body	
Manifestations	**Systematic Pathogenesis**
Aversion to cold, cold limbs relieved by warmth	Yang qi unable to move outward leading to poor warmth of the body
Pale face and tongue, deep slow pulse	Contraction of blood vessels leading to poor filling and nourishing of blood
Absence of sweat	Tightness of the muscular interstices
Loss of thirst, excessive clear urine	No impairment of body fluids
Constipation, pain and tenderness of the abdomen	Yin cold accumulating and obstructing qi flow
Loose stools	Disturbance of spleen yang and spleen qi leading to poor transportation and transformation

3. COMPARISON BETWEEN EXTERIOR AND INTERIOR PATTERNS

The major differences between exterior and interior patterns are associated with the location and manifestations of the disorder, the nature of the onset of the attack, and the duration and severity of the illness. The comparison is shown in Table 6.13.

Table 6.13 Comparison between Exterior and Interior Patterns

Properties	Exterior Pattern	Interior Pattern
Location	Exterior of the body	Interior of the body
Onset of attack	Sudden	Gradual

Duration of illness	Shorter	Longer
Manifestations	Chills accompanied by fever	Fever or aversion to cold
Tongue coating	Thin	Thick
Pulse condition	Floating	Deep
Severity of illness	Milder	More severe

4. HALF EXTERIOR-HALF INTERIOR PATTERNS

When the disorder is located in the area between the exterior and interior of the body the pattern type is termed a half exterior-half interior pattern.

General Overview

An overview of half exterior-half interior patterns is shown in Table 6.14.

Table 6.14 Half Exterior-Half Interior Patterns

Main Diagnostic Points	Pathogenesis	Pattern
Alternating attacks of fever and chills at irregular intervals	Body resistance (vital qi) and pathogenic factors (evil qi) fighting each other in the half exterior-half interior region of the body.	Shao yang
Alternating attacks of fever and chills at regular intervals		Malaria

Common Manifestations and Analysis of Half Exterior-Half Interior Patterns

Common manifestations and analyses of their pathogenesis are shown in Table 6.15.

Table 6.15 Manifestations and Analysis of Half Exterior-Half Interior Patterns

Common Pathogenesis	
Body resistance (vital qi) and pathogenic factors (evil qi) fighting each other in the half exterior-half interior region of the body	
Manifestations	**Systematic Pathogenesis**
Alternating attacks of chills and fever	Chills occurring as pathogens enter; fever occurring as the struggle waxes
Fullness and distension of the chest and hypochondrium	Pathogens entering the shao yang channel leading to obstruction of qi in the channel
Poor appetite, nausea and vomiting	Stagnation of gallbladder qi leading to disturbance of stomach qi

Irritability	Upward stirring of heat affecting the mind
Bitter taste in mouth, dry mouth, dizziness	Gallbladder heat steaming upward
Wiry pulse	Stagnation of gallbladder qi

5. COLD PATTERNS

Patterns caused either directly by an attack of external cold or by yang deficiency leading to prosperity of yin are classified as cold patterns.

Common Pattern Types

Cold pattern types are clinically classified into exterior cold patterns and interior cold patterns. The latter includes deficiency cold patterns and excess cold patterns.

Common Manifestations and Pathogenesis of Cold Patterns

Common manifestations for cold patterns and their pathogenesis are shown in Table 6.16.

Table 6.16 Manifestations and Pathogenesis of Cold Patterns

Property	Manifestations	Pathogenesis
Cold	Chills; aversion to cold; preference for warmth; cold limbs; pain with sensation of cold in the lumbar region, back, abdomen, or legs	Pathogenic cold suppressing yang qi, or insufficiency of yang qi leading to poor warmth of the body
Pale, clear, or white	Pale face; pale tongue and lips; white tongue coating; white sputum; or clear urine	Pathogenic cold suppressing yang qi, or insufficiency of yang qi leading to poor promotion of blood circulation
Hypoactive	Desire to lie down; listlessness; lassitude; preference for quiet environments; no desire to speak; dull expression; slow pulse	Cold suppressing yang qi, or yang qi deficiency leading to poor promotion of vitality
Thin, clear	Thin sputum; thin saliva; thin nasal discharge; thin pus; thin vaginal discharge; or thin stools	Cold, without damage to the body fluids
Moist	Moist tongue coating; absence of thirst; no dry sensation in the nose or mouth	Cold, without damage to the body fluids

Analysis of Etiology and Pathogenesis

The analysis of the etiology and pathogenesis of cold patterns is shown in Table 6.17.

Table 6.17 Etiology and Pathogenesis of Cold Patterns

Comparison of Cold Patterns

Cold patterns are classified into exterior, interior, deficiency, or excess types. The pathogenesis and main points for differential diagnosis are shown in Table 6.18.

Table 6.18 Comparison of Cold Patterns

Pattern		Pathogenesis	Main points
Exterior cold		Wind cold attacking exterior of the body	Sudden attack, shorter illness duration
Interior cold	Deficiency cold	Constitutional yang deficiency or consumption of yang qi leading to poor warmth	Weak constitution, longer illness process
	Excess cold	Cold directly attacking inside of the body, or overeating of cold and raw food and drink	Sudden attack, shorter illness process

Diagnosis in Traditional Chinese Medicine

6. HEAT PATTERNS

Patterns caused by external heat, by overeating of pungent and hot food, by extreme exposure to one of the seven emotions (grief, joy, anger, anxiety/melancholy, and fear/fright) or by yin deficiency leading to deficiency heat are classified as heat patterns.

Common Pattern Types

Common pattern types are clinically classified as either exterior heat patterns or interior heat patterns. The latter includes deficiency heat patterns as well as excess heat patterns.

Common Manifestations and Pathogenesis for Heat Patterns

Common manifestations for heat patterns and their pathogenesis are shown in Table 6.19.

Table 6.19 Manifestations and Pathogenesis for Heat Patterns

Main Diagnostic Points	Manifestations	Pathogenesis
Heat	High fever, tidal fever, low-grade fever, five-palm heat, malar flush or red zygomatic region, red tongue or redness of the affected area	Excess heat, or insufficiency of yin fluids producing deficiency heat, then steaming outward
Yellow/red	Yellow coloration of sputum, nasal discharge, vaginal discharge, stools, urine, or tongue coating; red tongue, red eyes, red, red lips, flushed face and red skin	Heat impairing body fluids; heat speeding up blood circulation
Hyperactive	Irritability, desire to move and speak, rapid pulse	Excess heat, or insufficiency of yin fluids producing upward stirring of deficiency heat
Thick, sticky	Thick sputum, nasal discharge, vaginal discharge, dark and scant urine, dry mouth, throat, nose, or tongue without salivation, dry stools	Heat impairing body fluids
Dry	Dry mouth, throat, nose, or tongue without salivation, dry stools	Heat impairing body fluids

Analysis of Etiology and Pathogenesis of Cold Patterns

An analysis of the etiology and pathogenesis of cold patterns is shown in Table 6.20.

Table 6.20 Etiology and Pathogenesis of Heat Patterns

External heat attack
Constitutional heat
Emotional distress
Consumption of yin fluids due to lingering illness
Indulgence in sexual activity
Severe diarrhea, sweating, or vomiting

→ Production of internal heat →

Flaring up
Steaming out
Impairment of yin fluids

→ Heat pattern →

Stirring of internal heat →
Powerful blood circulation
Hyperfunction of the internal organs
→ Fever, red tongue or redness of the affected area and rapid pulse

Steaming out of yin fluids → Yellow and thick secretions or excretions
Impairment of yin fluids → Poor moistening
→ Dry mouth, nose or tongue without salivation and dry stools

Comparison of Different Heat Patterns

Heat patterns are classified into exterior, interior, deficiency, and excess types. Their pathogenesis and main points for differential diagnosis are shown in Table 6.21.

Table 6.21 Comparison of Different Heat Patterns

Pattern		Pathogenesis	Main points
Exterior heat		Wind heat attacking the exterior of the body	Sudden attack, short illness process
Interior Heat	Deficiency heat	Constitutional yin deficiency, or consumption of yin fluids producing deficiency heat	Weak constitution, longer illness process
	Excess heat	Constitutional heat, or pathogenic heat attack, or overeating of pungent and hot food	Sudden attack, shorter illness process

7. COMPARISON BETWEEN COLD PATTERNS AND HEAT PATTERNS

The main differences between cold patterns and heat patterns are seen in the manifestation of temperature aversion or preference, complexion, sweating, thirst, defecation, urination, tongue, and pulse conditions. The comparison is shown in Table 6.22.

Table 6.22 Comparison between Cold Patterns and Heat Patterns

Main Diagnostic Points	Cold Pattern	Heat Pattern
Aversion	Cold	Heat
Preference	Warming	Cooling
Complexion	Pale face	Flushed face
Thirst	Absence of thirst	Thirst
Limbs	Cold	Warm
Mental state	Listless	Irritability
Stools	Loose	Dry
Urine	Clear and massive	Dark and scant
Tongue condition	Pale tongue, white coating	Red tongue, yellow coating
Pulse condition	Slow	Rapid

8. DEFICIENCY PATTERNS

Deficiency patterns are caused by a weakness of vital qi, which is often the result of a weak constitution or due to chronic illness.

Common Pattern Types

Common pattern types include qi deficiency pattern, blood deficiency pattern, yin deficiency pattern and yang deficiency pattern.

Common Manifestations and Pathogenesis of Deficiency Patterns

Common manifestations and their pathogenesis are arranged in Table 6.23.

Table 6.23 Manifestations and Pathogenesis of Deficiency Patterns

Main Diagnostic Points	Manifestations	Pathogenesis
Weak	Flaccidity of the limbs, emaciation; shortness of breath, respirations, cough or asthma, sounding with a low voice, speaking in low voice, loose stools, urinary incontinence	Insufficiency of vital qi leading to poor promotion of qi, blood, and organ function
Pale	Pale face without moisture; pale, thick, and tender tongue	Insufficiency of vital qi leading to poor promotion of circulation of qi and blood
Sweating	Spontaneous sweating	Insufficiency of yang and qi leading to looseness in the exterior
	Night sweats	Insufficiency of yin producing deficiency heat and steaming sweat outward
Passive	Listlessness, lassitude, somnolence	Insufficiency of vital qi leading to poor promotion of vitality
Dry, dysphoric	Irritability, red zygomatic area, five-palm heat, dry mouth and throat, dry stools	Insufficiency of yin fluids leading to poor nourishment; upward stirring of deficiency heat affecting the mind
Forceless pulse	Weak pulse or thin, deep, or distinct pulse with forceless beating	Insufficiency of yang qi leading to poor promotion of blood circulation

Analysis of Etiology and Pathogenesis of Deficiency Patterns

An analysis of the etiology and pathogenesis of deficiency patterns is shown in Table 6.24.

Table 6.24 Etiology and Pathogenesis Deficiency Patterns

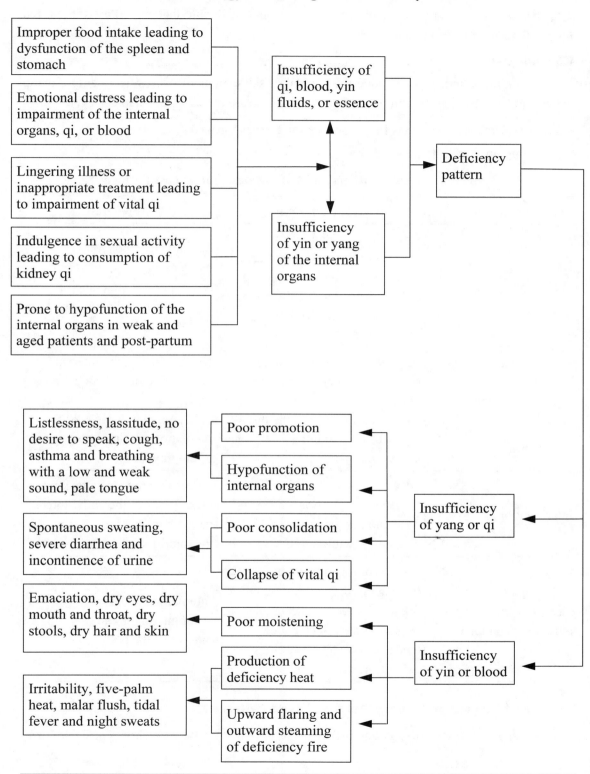

Improper food intake leading to dysfunction of the spleen and stomach

Emotional distress leading to impairment of the internal organs, qi, or blood

Lingering illness or inappropriate treatment leading to impairment of vital qi

Indulgence in sexual activity leading to consumption of kidney qi

Prone to hypofunction of the internal organs in weak and aged patients and post-partum

Insufficiency of qi, blood, yin fluids, or essence

Insufficiency of yin or yang of the internal organs

Deficiency pattern

Listlessness, lassitude, no desire to speak, cough, asthma and breathing with a low and weak sound, pale tongue

Poor promotion

Hypofunction of internal organs

Spontaneous sweating, severe diarrhea and incontinence of urine

Poor consolidation

Collapse of vital qi

Insufficiency of yang or qi

Emaciation, dry eyes, dry mouth and throat, dry stools, dry hair and skin

Poor moistening

Production of deficiency heat

Irritability, five-palm heat, malar flush, tidal fever and night sweats

Upward flaring and outward steaming of deficiency fire

Insufficiency of yin or blood

Chapter Six: Pattern Identification According to the Eight Principles

Table 6.24 Etiology and Pathogenesis Deficiency Patterns

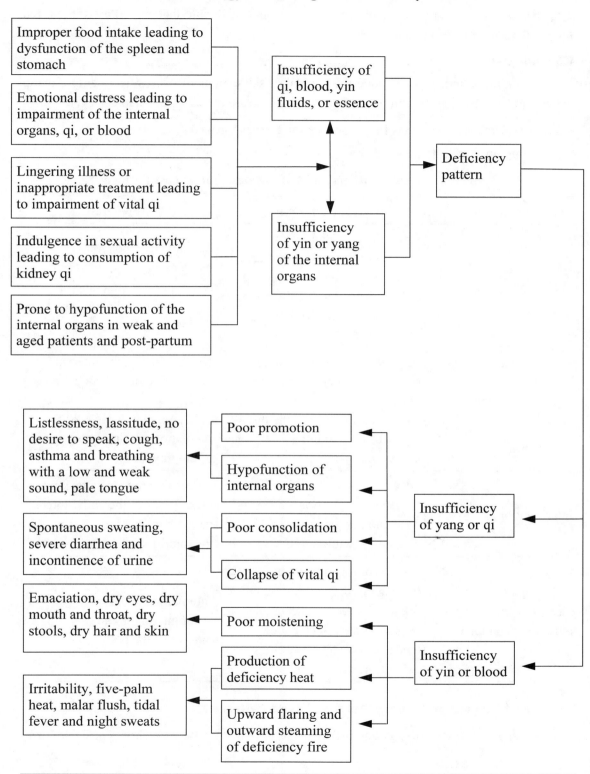

Chapter Six: Pattern Identification According to the Eight Principles   143

9. EXCESS PATTERNS

Excess patterns are caused by the prevalence of pathogenic factors and are more often seen in the earlier stages of a disease.

Common Pattern Types

Common pattern types include the clinical classifications of excess heat pattern, damp pattern, phlegm pattern, and blood stasis pattern. These are reviewed in Chapter Seven.

Common Manifestations and Pathogenesis for Excess Patterns

Common manifestations for excess patterns are shown in Table 6.25.

Table 6.25 Manifestations and Pathogenesis for Excess Patterns

Main Diagnostic Points	Manifestations	Pathogenesis
Inspection	Irritability; sudden loss of consciousness; delirium; flushed face; bloodshot eyes; tight and puffy tongue with thick yellow coating; thick and yellow secretions and excretions	Pathogenic wind, cold, summerheat, dryness, fire, toxins or insect bites attacking the body, causing vital qi to rise against invading pathogens
Auscultation and olfaction	Speaking, breathing, coughing, and asthma sounding in a high voice; excessive sputum with wheezing sound from the throat; heavy or foul-smelling secretions and excretions	Dysfunction of the internal organs leading to production of phlegm, phlegm fluids, water qi, damp, blood stasis, or food stagnation causing obstruction of the flow of qi
Interrogation	Fever, aversion to heat; constipation; dysuria; severe distension or pain; persistent discomfort without relief	External pathogens attacking the exterior of the body; internal pathogens accumulating in the interior of the body
Palpation and pulse examination	Replete pulse with forceful beating or wiry and rolling pulse; fullness, distension, accumulation, or pain of the affected area; tenderness, redness, swelling, or pain of the affected area	Internal pathogens accumulating in the interior of the body

Analysis of Etiology and Pathogenesis for Excess Patterns

An analysis of the etiology and pathogenesis for excess patterns is shown in Table 6.26.

Table 6.26 Etiology and Pathogenesis for Excess Patterns

```
Attacks of external
pathogens including
six environmental        ──────────────►   Vital qi
and epidemic                               struggling
febrile pathogens                          against
                                           invading
                                           pathogens
Unclean food intake ──►  Accumulation of                          Excess
                         parasites                      ────►     pattern
Overeating of food  ──►  Stagnation of food
                                           Material
                         Stagnation of     pathogens
                    ──►   qi and blood  ─► obstructing
Dysfunction of the                         the interior
internal organs                            of the body
                         Retention of
                    ──►  damp, phlegm,
                         phlegm fluids,
                         and water qi
```

```
Flushed face, bloodshot eyes,
restlessness, mental confusion,     ◄──  Over promotion of
speaking, breathing, cough or            yang qi
asthma in high voice, fever,                                          Flaring up of
wiry and rolling pulse with         ◄──  Hyperfunction of the    ◄──  excess heat   ◄──
forceful beating                         internal organs

Thick yellow secretions or          ◄──  Consumption of yin
excretions                               fluids

Severe distending pain                   Qi stagnation
aggravated by pressure; wheez-
ing sound in the throat; olig-                                        Obstruction
uria; constipation; fullness of     ◄──                               caused by      ◄──
the chest or abdomen; tender-            Pathogens                    material
ness, redness, pain, and swell-          accumulating in              pathogens
ing in affected area; red and            zang or fu organs
shriveled tongue
```

10. COMPARISON OF DEFICIENCY AND EXCESS PATTERNS

The difference between deficiency patterns and excess patterns is most visible in the condition of the spirit, physical activity, manner of breathing and speaking, properties of pain, duration of illness, and tongue and pulse conditions. The comparison is shown in Table 6.27.

Table 6.27 Comparison of Deficiency and Excess Patterns

Pattern	Deficiency	Excess
Spirit	Listlessness	Excitement
Physical activity	Desire to lie down	Desire to move
Breathing and speaking	In low weak voice	In high voice
Pain	Dull	Severe
Illness process	Longer	Shorter
Tongue	Pale, thick, and tender	Tight and shriveled
Pulse	Weak	Replete
Quality of qi	Insufficient or collapsed	Sufficient or obstructed

11. YIN PATTERNS

Yin patterns are basically subdivided into the categories of interior patterns, cold patterns, and deficiency patterns, depending on their general properties.

Common Pattern Types

This section discusses only yin exhaustion patterns, as the other pattern types such as interior, deficiency, and cold patterns have previously been discussed.

Common Manifestations and Analysis of Yin Exhaustion Patterns

The common manifestations and analysis of the pathogenesis for yin exhaustion patterns are shown in Table 6.28.

Table 6.28 Common Manifestations and Analysis of Yin Exhaustion Patterns

Etiology	General Pathogenesis	Common Pathogenesis	Manifestations
Long-lasting illness	Severe impairment of yin fluids leading to yin exhaustion	Gradual consumption of body fluids	Oily, sticky, warm, and salty sweating, thirst with desire for cold drinks
High fever with profuse sweating		Sudden loss of body fluids	Warm limbs, irritability, aversion to heat, red tongue without moisture, flooding rapid pulse with forceless beating
Severe vomiting, diarrhea, or bleeding			

12. Yang Patterns

Yang patterns are basically subdivided into the categories of exterior patterns, heat patterns, and excess patterns, depending on their general properties.

Common Pattern Types

This section only discusses yang exhaustion patterns, as the other pattern types such as exterior, excess, and heat patterns have previously been discussed.

Common Manifestations and Analysis of Yang Exhaustion Patterns

The common manifestations and analysis of the pathogenesis for yang exhaustion patterns are shown in Table 6.29.

Table 6.29 Common Manifestations and Analysis Yang Exhaustion Patterns

Etiology	Common Pathogenesis	Systematic Pathogenesis	Manifestations
Long-lasting illness	Severe impairment of yang qi leading to yang exhaustion	Gradual consumption of yang qi	Shortness of breath, pale face, indistinct pulse
Inappropriate treatment such as inducing severe sweating, vomiting or diarrhea		Sudden loss of yang qi	Profuse sweating
Yin exhaustion		Poor warmth of the limbs and body	Cold sweats, cold limbs, lack of thirst or desire for hot drinks, pale moist tongue
		Poor control of yin fluid leading to yang qi floating away	

13. Comparison of Yin and Yang Exhaustion Patterns

The difference between yin exhaustion patterns and yang exhaustion patterns is most visible in the body temperature in the limbs and skin, the complexion, sweating, thirst, urination, and condition of the pulse. The comparison is shown in Table 6.30.

Table 6.30 Comparison of Yin and Yang Exhaustion Patterns

Pattern	Yin Exhaustion	Yang Exhaustion
Limbs	Warm	Cold
Skin	Warm, dry	Cold, moist

Complexion	Malar flush	Sudden paleness
Sweat	Warm, salty, sticky, and oily	Profuse, cold
Thirst	Thirst with desire for cold drinks	Lack of thirst or desire for hot drinks
Urine	Scant	Scant
Pulse condition	Thin rapid pulse at the early stage; swift or even indistinct pulse at the late stage	Floating rapid pulse with forceless beating at the early stage; feeble or even indistinct pulse at the late stage

14. MAIN POINTS FOR ATTENTION IN YIN AND YANG EXHAUSTION PATTERNS

Scant urine can be found in both yin and yang exhaustion patterns, but the pathogenesis is different. The comparison is shown in Table 6.31.

Table 6.31 Comparison of Yin and Yang Exhaustion Patterns

Pattern	Urine Amount	Pathogenesis
Yin exhaustion	Scant	Insufficiency of body fluids leading to a lack of source for urine
Yang exhaustion	Scant	Dysfunction of the kidney leading to impaired opening and closing of the bladder

The pulse conditions in yin and yang exhaustion patterns differ from each other. In addition, they differ at different stages of each pattern. This is shown in Table 6.32.

Table 6.32 Comparison of Pulse Conditions in Yin and Yang Exhaustion Patterns

Pattern	Stage	Pulse Condition	Pathogenesis
Yin Exhaustion	Early stage	Thin and rapid	Yin collapse leading to yin qi losing its attachment and flowing outward
	Late stage	Swift or indistinct	Yin collapse leading to poor filling of the blood vessels
Yang Exhaustion	Early stage	Floating and rapid with forceless beat	Yang collapse leading to yang qi flowing outward
	Late stage	Indistinct	Yang collapse leading to poor promotion of blood circulation

III. RELATIONSHIP OF PATTERNS ACCORDING TO THE EIGHT PRINCIPLES

There are various relationships among the patterns classified according to the eight principles. These include transmission, true or false presentation, and simultaneously occurring patterns.

1. TRANSMISSION OF PATTERNS

All patterns classified under the eight principles can transform into another in certain conditions which are determined by the state of vital qi and by pathogenic factors. In clinical practice, a transmission between patterns mainly occurs between exterior and interior patterns, cold and heat patterns, and deficiency and excess patterns (see Tables 6.33 to 6.35).

Table 6.33 Transmission Occurring between Exterior and Interior Patterns

Transmission	Process	Characteristics
Exterior pathogens entering the interior of the body	Exterior pattern occurs first, followed by interior pattern	Exterior pattern disappears when interior pattern appears
Interior pathogens being transmitted outward	After sweating, high fever, severe thirst, and irritability have been relieved; after measles, fever, asthma, cough, and irritability have been relieved; after jaundice, distending pain of the hypochondrium, fever, and vomiting have been relieved.	Interior pattern becoming milder

Table 6.34 Transmission Occurring Between Heat and Cold Patterns

Transmission	Process	Characteristics
Cold pattern into heat pattern	Cold pattern occurs first, followed by heat pattern	Cold pattern disappears when heat pattern appears
Heat pattern into cold pattern	Heat pattern occurs first, followed by cold pattern	Heat pattern disappears when cold pattern appears

Table 6.35 Transmission Occurring between Deficiency and Excess Patterns

Transmission	Process	Characteristics
Excess pattern into deficiency pattern[3]	Excess pattern occurs first, followed by deficiency pattern	Excess pattern disappears when deficiency pattern appears
Deficiency pattern into excess pattern	With proper treatment, nursing, and health care, vital qi becomes stronger until it manifests as excess symptoms	Deficiency pattern disappears when excess manifestations appear

---

[3] There are two forms of excess patterns transferring into deficiency patterns, shown in Table 6.36.

Table 6.36 Excess Patterns Transferring into Deficiency Patterns

Type		Manifestations	Pathogenesis
Type One	Early stage	Excess pattern	Vital qi is adequate to stand up to the invasion of pathogenic factors
	Late stage	Deficiency pattern	Difficult or long-lasting illness has impaired vital qi
Type Two		Deficiency pattern following profuse sweating, severe diarrhea, and vomiting	Inappropriate treatment such as powerful diaphoretics, drastic purgatives, or emetic drugs has damaged vital qi

2. True or False Manifestations of Patterns

Sometimes, false manifestations will appear when a pattern reaches its extreme. True or false manifestations of patterns most often occur in heat and cold patterns and as well in excess and deficiency patterns (see Table 6.37). Keys to identifying a true manifestation from a false manifestation include the following:

- True manifestations always appear before false manifestations.
- False manifestations do not appear until true manifestations reach their extreme.
- True manifestations still exist after false manifestations occur.
- The tongue and pulse condition always support the diagnosis of a true manifestation.

Table 6.37 True or False Manifestations of a Pattern

Pattern	Process	Pathogenesis
Heat pattern with false cold manifestations	Heat manifestations appear before cold manifestations; cold manifestations occur when extreme heat flares up in the body; heat pattern still exists when cold manifestations appear	Excess internal yang keeping yin outside
Cold pattern with false heat manifestations	Cold manifestations appear before heat manifestations; heat manifestations occur when extreme cold accumulates in the body; cold pattern still exists when heat manifestations appear	Excess internal yin keeping yang outside
Excess pattern with false deficiency manifestations	Excess manifestations appear before deficiency manifestations; deficiency manifestations can be found in an excess pattern; excess pattern still exists when deficiency manifestations appear	Extreme excess appearing as deficiency manifestations
Deficiency pattern with false excess manifestations	Deficiency manifestations appear before excess manifestations; excess manifestations can be found in a deficiency pattern; deficiency pattern still exists when excess manifestations appear	Extreme deficiency appearing as excess manifestations

3. SIMULTANEOUS OCCURRENCE OF TWO PATTERNS

The simultaneous occurrence of two patterns is mainly found in the exterior and interior or upper and lower areas of the body. In other words, cold and heat manifestations can be found simultaneously in a single case, but in different locations of the body.

Exterior Cold-Interior Heat Pattern

Exterior cold-interior heat pattern refers to a combined pattern in which there are cold manifestations on the exterior of the body and manifestations in the interior (see Table 6.38).

Table 6.38 Exterior Cold-Interior Heat Pattern

Pattern	Examples	Pathogenesis
Exterior cold	Chills, headaches, absence of sweating, aching	External cold entering the interior of the body and producing heat; wind cold attacking the body and presenting as heat
Interior heat	Dysphoria, thirst, dry stools, scant dark urine	

Exterior Heat-Interior Cold Pattern

Exterior heat-interior cold pattern refers to a combined pattern in which there are heat manifestations on the exterior of the body and cold manifestations in the interior (see Table 6.39).

Table 6.39 Exterior Heat-Interior Cold Pattern

Pattern	Examples	Pathogenesis
Exterior heat	Fevers, chills, headaches, sore throat, and coughing	Inappropriate treatment such as purgation damaging spleen yang when external heat attacks; wind heat attacking the body, presenting as cold
Interior cold	Abdominal pain, preference for warmth and pressure, loose stools, excessive clear urine	

Heat Pattern in the Upper Body with Cold Pattern in the Lower Body

This is a combined pattern in which there are heat manifestations occurring in the upper body, while cold manifestations are seen in the lower areas, as shown in Table 6.40.

Table 6.40 Heat Pattern in the Upper Body with Cold Pattern in the Lower Body

Pattern	Examples	Pathogenesis
Heat pattern in the upper area of the body	Fullness and feverishness of the chest and upper abdomen, dry throat, sore throat	Yang heat rising in the upper body while yin cold accumulates in the lower body
Cold pattern in the lower area of the body	Pain of the abdomen with preference for warmth and pressure, loose stools, clear urine	

Cold Pattern in the Upper Body with Heat Pattern in the Lower Body

This is a combined pattern in which there are cold manifestations occurring in the upper body, while heat manifestations occur in the lower body, as shown in the example given in Table 6.41.

Table 6.41 Cold Pattern in the Upper Body with Heat Pattern in the Lower Body

Pattern	Examples	Pathogenesis
Cold pattern in the upper area of the body	Pain of the upper abdomen with cold sensation, drooling with clear saliva	Yin cold obstructing the upper body with yang heat accumulating in the lower body
Heat pattern in the lower area of the body	Frequent, urgent and painful urination, scant dark urine	

Pattern Identification According to Pathogenic Factors

When applying this method of pattern identification, the practitioner takes the properties of pathogenic factors as guiding principles in order to analyze the manifestations obtained from the four diagnostic methods and then identify the pattern.

I. PATHOGENIC FACTORS

Pathogenic factors are clinically categorized into four groups:

- *External pathogenic factors*

  The six environmental phenomena, namely wind, cold, summerheat, dampness, dryness, and fire.

- *Internal pathogenic factors*

  Internal pathogenic factors include the seven emotions (grief, joy, anger, anxiety/melancholy, and fear/fright) as well as dysfunctions of qi, blood, or the internal organs such as qi deficiency, heart yin deficiency, and liver yang rising.

- *Pathogenic factors which are neither external nor internal*

  Pathogenic factors which are neither external nor internal include parasites, traumatic injury, improper food intake, insect bites, snakebites, overworking or overexertion, and indulgence in alcohol, drugs, or sexual activity.

- *Other pathogenic factors*

  Other pathogenic factors are those conditions produced by a prior disorder which then lead to subsequent disorders such as internal damp, phlegm, phlegm fluids, water qi, or blood stasis.

II. PATTERNS

Common patterns that will be discussed in this chapter arise from the six environmental phenomena, toxins, improper food intake, or phlegm. Others will be explained in Chapter Eight, "Pattern Identification According to Qi and Blood," and Chapter Nine, "Pattern Identification According to the Internal Organs."

1. WIND

Wind patterns are classified according to two groups: exterior wind and interior wind. Interior wind, known as liver wind, can be induced by extreme heat, liver yang rising, liver blood deficiency, or liver yin deficiency, and will be discussed in Chapter Nine, "Pattern Identification According to the Internal Organs." Exterior wind refers to pathogenic wind from the external environment. Only exterior wind patterns will be examined in Table 7.1.

Table 7.1 Exterior Wind Patterns

Manifestations	Pathogenesis	Clinical Pattern
Chills, low-grade fever, possibly skin rashes, itching, white thin tongue coating, floating moderate pulse	Wind attacking the exterior of the body leading to irregular opening and closing of the muscular interstices	Exterior deficiency
Cough, stuffy nose, sneezing, itching of the throat or sore throat, white thin tongue coating, floating pulse	Wind attacking the lung leading to dysfunction of the lung in dispersing and precipitating.	Wind attacking the lung
Sudden numbness and deviation of the eyes and the mouth; stiffness of the neck, clenched teeth, possibly spasms of the body and limbs	Wind attacking the channels and network vessels leading to qi stagnation	Wind attacking the network vessels
Migrating pain of the joints	Wind combining with cold damp and obstructing the channels and network vessels, affecting the joints	Wind impediment (bi)
Skin rashes and other skin lesions with itching	Wind attacking the skin and remaining in the muscular interstices	Wind attacking the skin

2. COLD

Cold patterns are clinically classified as either externally attacking cold or internally generated cold. The latter is caused by yang deficiency. As a deficiency pattern, internally-generated cold will be reviewed in Chapter Nine, "Pattern Identification According to the Internal Organs." Externally attacking cold is from an invasion of pathogenic cold caused by such activities as being caught in the rain, bathing in cold water, under-dressing for the weather, sleeping in cool air, or overindulging in raw and cold food and drinks, circumstances that restrain yang qi inside the body. Therefore, such conditions are identified as excess cold patterns, a category which includes both exterior cold patterns and interior cold patterns (see

Table 7.2). The former are caused by external cold attacking the exterior of the body; the latter are due to external cold attacking the internal organs or the qi and blood circulatory systems.

Table 7.2 Exterior and Interior Cold Patterns

Manifestations	Pathogenesis	Clinical Pattern
Chills possibly accompanied by low-grade fevers, headache, aching, lack of sweating, stuffy or runny nose, white thin tongue coating, floating tense pulse; or fixed pain in the joints with cold sensation	Wind cold invading and remaining in the muscular interstices, fighting with wei qi on the exterior of the body	Exterior cold; cold impediment
Aversion to cold, cold limbs, pain with cold sensation in local areas relieved by warmth, vomiting, diarrhea, cough, asthma, spitting of white sputum and saliva, pale facial complexion, white tongue coating, deep slow pulse with forceful beat	Pathogenic cold attacking and accumulating in the qi and blood circulatory systems and in the internal organs, impairing and restricting yang qi	Interior cold

3. SUMMERHEAT

Pathogenic summerheat is characterized by properties similar to fire and heat patterns, but is remarkably seasonal, so there are some differences in pathogenesis and manifestations.

Table 7.3 Summerheat Patterns

Manifestations	Pathogenesis	Clinical Pattern
Aversion to heat, profuse sweating, thirst with desire for drinks, shortness of breath, lassitude, listlessness, scant dark urine, red tongue, rapid pulse with forceless heat	Summerheat invading and accumulating in the body leading to impairment of both qi and body fluids	Summerheat
Low-grade or tidal fever, oppression in the chest, abdominal pain, nausea, lack of sweating, greasy tongue coating, soft pulse	Summerheat and dampness accumulating in the body leading to qi stagnation	Summerheat damp
High fever, possibly delirium, loss of consciousness, tension and convulsion of limbs	Upward stirring of extreme summerheat affecting the mind	Summerheat stroke

4. DAMPNESS

Dampness may occur in two ways. One is caused by external dampness attacking the body, affecting the exterior or interior of the body. The other type is caused by a dysfunction of the spleen in transporting and transforming dampness. The patterns discussed here fall into the category of exterior damp patterns (see Table 7.4). Patterns caused by internally-generated dampness, including damp heat and cold damp, will be examined below in Chapter Nine, "Pattern Identification According to the Internal Organs."

Table 7.4 Damp Patterns

Manifestations	Pathogenesis	Clinical Pattern
Heaviness of the head, or possibly soreness and pain of the whole body; or skin wetrashes with itching, chills, or chronic low-grade or tidal fever	External dampness due to living in a wet place or getting wet in the rain and fog, leading to damp accumulating on the exterior of the body and obstructing qi in the channels and network vessels	Exterior damp
Heaviness and pain of the joints, with limited range of motion	Dampness remaining in the joints and obstructing qi in the channels and network vessels	Damp impediment
Heaviness of the whole body, distension and fullness of the chest and upper abdomen, poor appetite, nausea, vomiting, diarrhea	Consumption of raw, cold, or unclean food or drinks causing the obstruction of spleen and stomach qi, leading to poor promotion of digestion	Dampness attacking the interior

5. DRYNESS

Dryness is divided into externally-attacking dryness and internally-generated dryness. Dryness patterns are clinically classified into internal dryness patterns and exterior dryness patterns. The former is caused by an insufficiency of blood or yin fluids leading to poor nourishment of the body. It will be discussed below in Chapter Eight, "Pattern Identification According to the Internal Organs." External dryness patterns are caused by pathogenic dryness attacking the exterior of the body and impairing body fluids. They are examined here in Table 7.5.

Table 7.5 Exterior Dryness Patterns

Manifestations	Pathogenesis	Clinical Pattern
Dry, possibly chapped skin, desquamation, dry mouth, lips, nose. and throat, yellow thin tongue coating, floating pulse	Dryness invading the exterior of the body	Dryness attacking the exterior

Dry cough or cough with scant sticky sputum, difficult expectoration, dry mouth, lips, and throat, dry stools, dry yellow thin tongue coating, floating pulse	Pathogenic dryness invading the lung and damaging lung yin	Dryness attacking the lung

6. FIRE

In TCM theory, extreme warm is classified as heat, and extreme heat as fire. Fire is clinically divided into externally-attacking fire and internally-generated fire. The former is due to an attack of external pathogenic fire, caused by living and working in locations with high temperatures, by epidemic febrile pathogens, by overeating of pungent and hot food causing the production of internal fire, or by long-lasting cold damp producing heat. Patterns caused by the above-listed factors are classified as excess fire patterns and include patterns of exterior heat, interior heat, and heat penetrating the pericardium. (See Table 7.6.) Internally-generated fire is caused by the chronic retention of internal pathogens such as cold, damp, phlegm, or phlegm fluids producing heat, by emotional distress inducing fire, or by a hyper-function of the internal organs brought about by fire. These are identified as excess fire patterns. In addition, conditions brought on by a yin deficiency producing fire are identified as deficiency fire patterns. Both of these types of internally-generated fire will be examined below in the Chapter Nine, "Pattern Identification According to the Internal Organs."

Table 7.6 Excess Fire Patterns

Manifestations	Pathogenesis	Clinical Pattern
Fever greater than chills, sore throat, yellow thin tongue coating, rapid floating pulse; or painful joints with redness, swelling, and hot sensation	Fire attacking the exterior of the body	Exterior heat; heat impediment
Fever, flushed face, aversion to heat, irritability, thirst with desire for cold drinks, dark scant urine, constipation, yellow tongue coating, flooding rolling rapid pulse	Upward stirring of fire impairing the body fluids	Interior fire
Fever, irritability, nose and gum bleeding, bruises on the skin, possibly expectoration of blood	Fire compressing the blood and forcing it out of the blood vessels	Bleeding
High fever, flushed face, irritability, mental confusion, delirium, possibly loss of consciousness	Extreme fire penetrating the pericardium and stirring upward affecting the mind	Fire penetrating the pericardium

7. TOXINS

Toxins refer to a variety of different factors which are shown in Table 7.7.

Table 7.7 Toxin Patterns

Toxin	Manifestations	Example
Epidemic pathogens	Sudden onset, severe reaction of the whole body, with infectious properties	Plague, hemorrhagic fever, chicken pox, German measles, diphtheria
Toxicity	Severe reaction of the whole body following snake and insect bites, erroneous intake of drugs or food	Poisoning due to snake and insect venom; drug or food poisoning; carbon monoxide poisoning
Six external pathogens in the extreme	Abnormally severe manifestations of the patterns caused by the six external pathogens	Tetanus (toxic wind attacking the channels and network vessels; unhealed skin ulcers (toxic damp obstructing the channels and network vessels)
Pathogens that cause severe external diseases	Severe redness, swelling, pain with hot sensation in the affected area, chronic unhealed ulcers	Sores, boils, abscesses, carbuncles, furuncles, ulcers, fistulas and gangrenes, tuberculosis of the bones and joints

8. FOOD STAGNATION

Food stagnation can be caused by improper food intake as well as by a dysfunction of the spleen and stomach in transforming, transporting, and digesting food that leads to undigested food remaining in the stomach and large intestine (see Table 7.8).

Table 7.8 Food Stagnation Patterns

Manifestations	Pathogenesis	Clinical Pattern
History of improper food intake followed by distension, fullness, and pain of the upper abdomen, loss of appetite, acid reflux, belching, nausea, vomiting, foul stools, thick greasy tongue coating, rolling pulse with forceful beat	Food stagnation leading to stagnation of stomach qi	Food stagnation
History of chronic indigestion, distension, fullness and discomfort of the upper abdomen, loss of appetite, pale face, lassitude, listlessness, loose stools containing undigested food, rolling pulse with forceless beat	Spleen qi deficiency leading to poor transportation and transformation of foodstuff	Spleen deficiency-food stagnation

9. Phlegm, Phlegm Fluids, and Water Qi

Phlegm, phlegm fluids, and water qi are special forms of dampness that are retained in the body. They are due to pathological changes caused by an accumulation of body fluids. At the same time, they are also pathogenic factors themselves. Phlegm, characterized by a thick and sticky quality, tends to accumulate in the lung or in localized areas of the body. Phlegm fluids, characterized by a thin and clear quality, tend to accumulate in any organ with a cavity such as the lung, pericardium, or stomach. Water qi, being water-like, may be retained in the muscles and subcutaneous tissues, a condition known as edema.

Phlegm

Compared to phlegm fluids, phlegm is of a thicker consistency and tends to accumulate in the lung, joints, tendons, channels, and network vessels. Phlegm patterns are discussed in Table 7.9.

Table 7.9 Phlegm Patterns

Manifestations	Pathogenesis	Clinical Pattern
Cough with thick and sticky sputum, oppression of the chest, greasy tongue coating, rolling pulse	Phlegm retained in the lung leading to reversal of lung qi	Lung disorders
Distension and fullness of the upper abdomen, nausea, expectoration of sticky saliva, poor appetite, greasy tongue coating, rolling pulse	Phlegm retained in the middle burner leading to reversal of stomach qi	Stomach disorders
Obesity, heaviness of the head, fuzzy thoughts, possibly loss of consciousness or epileptic seizures, depressive psychosis, mania	Upward stirring of phlegm disturbing the opening of the heart and misting the mind	Wind stroke; upward stirring of wind phlegm affecting the mind; upward flaring of phlegm fire misting the mind
Scrofula, goiter, subcutaneous nodules, plum pit sensation in throat	Phlegm accumulating in localized area	Phlegm accumulation

Phlegm Fluids

Phlegm fluid is a clear pathogen of a thin consistency which lodges in any body cavities, such as the chest or the abdomen. Phlegm fluids patterns are discussed in Table 7.10.

Table 7.10 Phlegm Fluids Patterns

Manifestations	Pathogenesis	Clinical Pattern
Cough, asthma with copious clear thin sputum, wheezing sound in throat, delicate tongue with white moist coating	Phlegm fluids retained in the lung leading to reversal of lung qi	Phlegm fluids retained in the lung
Distension and fullness of the upper abdomen, splashing sound in the abdomen, possibly expectoration of copious thin clear saliva	Phlegm fluids retained in the stomach and large intestine, leading to reversal of stomach qi	Phlegm fluids retained in the stomach
Stuffiness and fullness of the chest and hypochondrium, distending pain aggravated by breathing, coughing, and changing body position	Phlegm fluids retained in the chest and hypo-chondrium leading to stagnation of qi and blood	Phlegm fluids retained in the pericardium; phlegm fluids retained in the chest and hypochondrium

Water Qi

Water qi refers to a water-like pathogen. Combined with wind, it tends to attack the upper part of the body. Conditions of water qi which are caused by spleen or kidney yang qi deficiency will be examined here as shown in Table 7.11. Conditions which are brought about by a decline of heart and kidney yang, leading to water qi attacking the heart, will be discussed below in Chapter Nine, "Pattern Identification According to the Internal Organs."

Table 7.11 Water Qi Patterns

Manifestations	Pathogenesis	Clinical Pattern
Sudden onset of edema starting with the eyelids and face, then spreading to the trunk and limbs, chills, low-grade fever, white thin tongue coating, floating pulse	Wind attacking the lung leading to dysfunction of the lung in dredging the passage of water	Yang water (wind water attacking the lung)
Edema, cold limbs, poor appetite, distension of the abdomen, diarrhea, pale puffy tongue with white greasy tongue coating, weak rolling pulse	Spleen qi deficiency leading to dysfunction of the spleen in transporting and transforming damp, leading to water retention	Yin water (spleen yang qi deficiency)
Edema, cold limbs, soreness and weakness of the lumbar area and knees, scant urine, listlessness, lassitude, pale puffy tongue, weak deep pulse	Kidney qi deficiency causing dysfunction of the kidney in controlling the opening and closing of the bladder and leading to water retention	Yin water (kidney yang qi deficiency)

CHAPTER EIGHT

Pattern Identification According to Qi and Blood

Pattern identification according to qi and blood is a commonly used method for pattern identification which analyzes manifestations obtained from the four diagnostic methods by taking the healthy functioning and pathological characteristics of qi and blood as its guiding principles. This type of pattern identification is used for disorders without obvious cold or heat manifestations.

In clinical practice, common pattern types are classified into three basic groups. They are shown in Table 8.1.

Table 8.1 Common Qi and Blood Disorder Patterns

Qi Disorders	Blood Disorders	Combined Qi and Blood Disorders
Qi Deficiency Qi Fall Qi Stagnation Qi Reversal	Blood deficiency Blood stasis Blood heat Bleeding	Qi deficiency-blood deficiency Qi deficiency-blood stasis Qi-stagnation-blood stasis Qi failing to contain blood in vessels Qi collapse followed by blood collapse

I. PATTERNS ACCORDING TO QI

Common patterns in this category can be caused by a deficiency, falling, stagnation, or reversal (upward counterflow) of qi.

1. QI DEFICIENCY

Qi deficiency pattern causes poor functioning of the internal organs (See Table 8.2).

Table 8.2 Qi Deficiency Patterns

Common Pathogenesis	
Qi deficiency	
Manifestations	**Systematic Pathogenesis**
Lassitude, listlessness, shortness of breath, no desire to speak, low voice	Hypofunction of the internal organs leading to poor invigoration of the physical body and the vitality
Dizziness	Poor promotion of blood circulation to nourish the brain
Spontaneous sweating	Poor consolidation of the exterior
All manifestations aggravated after exercise	Exercise consuming qi
Pale or pink tongue	Inability to guide qi upward and nourish the tongue
Weak pulse	Poor promotion of blood circulating in the vessels

2. QI FALL

Qi fall refers to a condition based on the deficiency of qi marked by prolapse of the viscera. Qi fall patterns are discussed in Table 8.3.

Table 8.3 Qi Fall Patterns

Common Pathogenesis	
Qi deficiency	
Manifestations	**Systematic Pathogenesis**
Lassitude, listlessness, shortness of breath, no desire to speak, spontaneous sweating, pale tongue, weak pulse	Hypofunction of the internal organs, poor consolidation of the exterior of the body, and poor promotion of blood circulation
Prolapse of the uterus, rectum, stomach, and kidneys	Deficiency of spleen qi leading to inability to consolidate the internal organs

3. QI STAGNATION

In general, qi stagnation can be caused by emotional depression, improper food intake, an attack of external pathogens, sprain and contusion, or an obstruction by pathological by-products such as damp, phlegm, phlegm fluids, blood stasis, and stones. The qi stagnation patterns displayed in Table 8.4 are mainly brought about by emotional depression, which is closely related to liver qi stagnation.

Table 8.4 Qi Stagnation Patterns

Common Pathogenesis	
Liver qi stagnation	
Manifestations	**Systematic Pathogenesis**
Distending pain occurring in the chest, hypochondrium and abdominal region, frequent sighing	Qi flow stagnating in a localized area of the body
All manifestations aggravated or relieved by emotional changes	Qi flow becoming smoother as emotions improve, and vice versa
Wiry pulse	Qi flow stagnating in the blood vessels

4. QI REVERSAL

The formation of qi reversal is based on qi stagnation. Lung qi reversal can be caused by an attack of external pathogens or an accumulation of phlegm and phlegm fluids; stomach qi reversal commonly results from an accumulation of cold, heat, phlegm fluids, food stagnation, or blood stasis; liver qi reversal often arises from emotional depression, and possibly violent rage. Qi reversal patterns are discussed in Table 8.5.

Table 8.5 Qi Reversal Patterns

Manifestations	**Common Pathogenesis**	**Systematic Pathogenesis**
Cough, asthma, or breathing with difficulty and expectoration of sputum	Dysfunction of the lung in dispersing and descending	Reverting lung qi
Nausea, vomiting, belching, acid reflux and hiccups	Dysfunction of the stomach in regulating and precipitating	Reverting stomach qi
Headache, dizziness, vertigo, tinnitus, sighing, sudden loss of consciousness, or possibly expectoration of blood	Dysfunction of the liver in spreading and precipitating	Reverting liver qi

II. PATTERNS ACCORDING TO BLOOD

Common patterns related to blood disorders can be caused by a deficiency, stagnation, or heat in the blood level and bleeding.

1. BLOOD DEFICIENCY

Insufficiency of blood can be due either to the loss of blood or the poor production of blood. The former includes various kinds of bleeding, such as those caused by menorrhagia, emotinal distress, or a chronic illness that consumes blood. Blood deficiency due to a poor production of blood is caused by the factors such as dysfunction of the spleen and stomach in transforming and transporting and inadequate nutritional intake leading to a poor source of blood. Blood deficiency patterns are reviewed in Table 8.6.

Table 8.6 Blood Deficiency Patterns

Common Pathogenesis	
Blood deficiency	
Manifestations	**Systematic Pathogenesis**
Sallow complexion or pale face	Poor nourishment of the face
Dizziness	Poor nourishment of the brain
Pale lips and tongue	Poor nourishment of the lips and tongue
Numbness, pale nails	Poor nourishment of the body and extremities
Palpitations	Poor nourishment of the heart and spirit
Scant menstruation of a light color, delayed menstrual cycle, and possibly amenorrhea	Poor source of menstrual blood
Thin pulse	Poor filling of the blood vessels

2. BLOOD STASIS

Blood stasis can be caused by traumatic injury leading to bleeding, by qi stagnation leading to an obstruction of the blood circulation, by qi deficiency leading to poor promotion of blood circulation, by excess cold leading to a constriction of the blood vessels, or by excess heat or phlegm fire leading to an accumulation of blood. Blood stasis patterns are reviewed in Table 8.7.

Table 8.7 Blood Stasis Patterns

Common Pathogenesis	
Blood stagnation	
Manifestations	**Systematic Pathogenesis**
Stabbing pain fixed in the affected area	Obstructed flow of both qi and blood
Ecchymosis, petechia, bruises	Blood leaking out of the blood vessels, but retained in a localized area
Abdominal accumulations (inflammatory or non-inflammatory masses, tumors, or cancers)	Accumulation due to blood stasis

Diagnosis in Traditional Chinese Medicine

Scaly and dry skin, dusky face	Poor nourishment of the skin
Pain in the lower abdomen during menstruation, scant menstruation with blood clots	Obstructed menstruation
Purple tongue and choppy pulse	Obstructed flow of both qi and blood

Blood stasis is clinically classified into the four subcategories shown in Table 8.8.

Table 8.8 Blood Stasis Pattern Types

Pattern Types	Manifestations	Pathogenesis
Qi deficiency	Pale or sallow complexion, lassitude, listlessness, low voice and no desire to speak, spontaneous sweating, hemiparesis, stabbing pain, hemoptysis, no pulsation in the upper limbs or lower limbs, pale purple tongue or purple spots on tip or both sides of tongue	Qi deficiency leading to an inability to promote blood circulation
Qi stagnation	Irritability, sighing, accumulation in the hypochondrium without migration, abdominal masses, subcutaneous varicose veins in the abdominal wall, vascular spiders in the skin, dysmenorrhea with dark-colored menstruation, amenorrhea, and wiry choppy pulse	Liver qi stagnation leading to obstructed circulation of blood
Accumulation of excess cold	Cold limbs with pale or blue-green color in the skin, pain in the limbs and abdomen with cold sensation relieved by warmth, but aggravated by cold, delayed menstruation, or lack of circulation in the upper and lower limbs	Constriction of the blood vessels by accumulated cold leading to obstructed blood circulation
Accumulation of excess heat	Pain in the body or limbs relieved by cold; various skin infections marked by redness, swelling, hot sensation and pain in the affected area; abdominal pain, tenderness, irritability, constipation, scant dark urine, dark red tongue, rapid pulse	Excess heat accumulating in the blood vessels leading to an obstruction of the blood circulation

3. BLOOD HEAT

Blood heat pattern refers to a pattern occurring in the blood system and is marked by excess heat compressing the blood out of the vessels. Blood heat patterns are reviewed in Table 8.9.

Table 8.9 Blood Heat Patterns

Common Pathogenesis	
Excess blood heat	
Manifestations	**Systematic Pathogenesis**
Bleeding in various locations in large amounts and dark red in color	Excess heat damaging the blood vessels leading to extravascular bleeding
Irritability, insomnia	Excess heat stirring the mind
Thirst	Excess heat impairing yin fluids
Dark red tongue and wiry rapid pulse with forceful beat	Rapid circulation of blood and overfilling of the blood vessels

4. BLEEDING

Bleeding can be found in blood heat patterns, blood stasis patterns, qi deficiency patterns, and qi collapse patterns (see Table 8.10).

Table 8.10 Bleeding

Pattern	Characteristics of Bleeding	Complex Manifestations	Tongue Condition	Pulse Condition	Pathogenesis
Blood heat	Red, thick, and sticky	Fever, flushed face, thirst, irritability, constipation, dark scant urine	Red	Rapid	Excess heat damaging the blood vessels
Qi deficiency	Light red and thin	Pale face, poor appetite, loose stools, lassitude	Pale	Weak	Qi deficiency leading to dysfunction of the spleen in keeping blood in the vessels
Blood stasis	Dark red and thick, even with clots	Stabbing pain in fixed area, ecchymosis, petechia	Purple	Choppy	Stagnated blood obstructing the blood vessels, causing bleeding
Qi collapse	Heavy	Sudden paling of face, profuse cold sweat, cold limbs	Pale	Distinct	Qi collapse leading to yang exhaustion

III. PATTERN IDENTIFICATION FOR COMBINED QI–BLOOD DISORDERS

In some cases, a qi disorder may be combined with a blood disorder. The common patterns of qi-blood disorders are shown in Table 8.11.

Table 8.11 Qi-Blood Disorders

Pattern	Manifestations	Pathogenesis
Qi deficiency-blood deficiency	As seen in Tables 8.2 and 8.6	Qi deficiency leading to poor production of blood; blood deficiency leading to poor production of qi
Qi deficiency-blood stasis	As seen in Tables 8.2 and 8.7	Qi deficiency leading to obstruction of blood circulation
Qi-blood stagnation	As seen in Table 8.4 and 8.7	Qi stagnation leading to obstructed circulation of blood
Qi deficiency-bleeding	As seen in Tables 8.2 and 8.10	Spleen qi deficiency failing to keep blood circulating in the vessels
Bleeding→qi collapse →yang exhaustion	As seen in Tables 8.10 and 6.28	Qi collapse following blood collapse; yang exhaustion followed by qi collapse

Pattern Identification
According to the Internal Organs

The method of pattern identification which is based on internal organs theory and accordingly differentiated by the affected zang and fu organs is called pattern identification according to the internal organs. Pattern identification according to the internal organs uses the condition of the internal organs as the guiding principle, in order to pinpoint the location where the disorder occurs. This method of pattern identification is generally used to analyze interior patterns.

The main purpose and tasks of this type of pattern identification are to confirm the location where the disorder occurs. Once the disorder is located, a final diagnosis can be given.

A firm background knowledge of the physiological functions of each zang and fu organ, as well as the characteristics of pathological changes in each of them, are required in order to use this method of pattern identification.

I. PATTERNS ACCORDING TO THE LUNG

Pattern identification for disorders of the lung is based on understanding the physiological functions and pathological characteristics of the lung. The manifestations obtained from the four diagnostic methods are analyzed in this light and a final pattern diagnosis is achieved.

Lung disorders mainly involve the functions of the lung in governing respiration, water metabolism, and wei qi, and thus manifest as changes in cough, asthma, sputum, and sensations of the chest.

1. MAIN ANALYSIS OF DISORDERS OF THE LUNG

The common manifestations and pathogenesis for disorders of the lung are analyzed in Table 9.1.

Table 9.1 Analysis of Common Manifestations and Pathogenesis for the Lung

Manifestations	Common Pathogenesis	Systematic Pathogenesis
Cough, asthma	Dysfunction of the lung in governing qi and respiration	Dysfunction of the lung in dispersing and descending qi
Shortness of breath, no desire to speak, low voice		Insufficiency of pectoral qi[4] leading to inability to support speaking and breathing
Sputum	Dysfunction of the lung in governing the metabolism of the body fluids	Retention of body fluids leading to production of phlegm
Edema		Retention of body fluids in the skin and limbs
Pain in the chest	External pathogens attacking the lung	Obstruction of lung qi in the chest
Fullness and oppression of the chest		Obstruction of qi and blood flow
Coughing blood, nasal bleeding		Fire damaging the blood vessels of the lung

2. COMMON PATTERN TYPES

All patterns commonly seen in lung disorders are classified as either excess patterns or deficiency patterns. Deficiency patterns occur in chronic cases or involve other internal organs; excess patterns are caused by an attack of external pathogens or by phlegm retention.

Lung Qi Deficiency

This pattern refers to a condition in which the functions of the lung become weak in governing qi and defending against the attack of external pathogens (see Table 9.2).

Table 9.2 Lung Qi Deficiency

Common Pathogenesis	
Lung qi deficiency	
Manifestations	**Systematic Pathogenesis**
Cough with weak voice	Insufficiency of pectoral qi* leading to inability to support speaking and breathing
Shortness of breath or severe cough after exercising	Exercise that consumes qi

---

[4] Pectoral qi refers to ancestral qi. It consists of a combination of inhaled air and ying and wei qi that originate from foodstuff. Pectoral qi is located in the chest.

Thin and clear sputum	Qi deficiency leading to inability to distribute body fluids
No desire to speak, low voice	Speaking that consumes qi
Shallow and difficult breathing, lassitude, listlessness	Poor invigoration of the physical body and the vitality
Spontaneous sweating, aversion to wind	Poor consolidation of the exterior of the body
Pale face and tongue	Poor nourishment of blood in its upward circulation
Weak pulse	Poor promotion of blood circulation

Main manifestations: Cough, asthma with thin clear sputum, combined with manifestations as seen in **qi deficiency patterns (Table 8.2).**

Lung Yin Deficiency

This pattern is caused by lung yin deficiency leading to poor nourishment of the body and the production of deficiency heat (see Table 9.3).

Table 9.3 Lung Yin Deficiency

Common Pathogenesis	
Lung yin deficiency	
Manifestations	**Systematic Pathogenesis**
Dry cough or scant and sticky sputum with difficult expectoration	Deficiency fire impairing the body fluids
Bloody sputum or coughing blood	Deficiency fire damaging the lung collateral channels
Dry mouth and throat, thirst	Poor nourishment of the opening of the lung
Emaciation	Poor nourishment of the trunk and limbs
Tidal fever, five-palm heat	Deficiency fire steaming outward
Night sweats	Yang qi moving inwards during sleep, assisting deficiency heat, causing the body fluids to go out
Malar flush, irritability	Stirring of deficiency fire
Red tongue with or without scant coating, thin rapid pulse	Deficiency fire accumulating in the body
Dry cough or scant and sticky sputum with difficult expectoration	Deficiency fire impairing the body fluids

Main manifestations: Dry cough or cough with scant sputum, combined with manifestations as seen in **yin deficiency patterns (Table 6.10).**

Wind Heat Attacking the Lung

This pattern is caused by wind heat attacking the lung leading to a dysfunction of the lung in dispersing and precipitating qi (see Table 9.4).

Table 9.4 Wind Heat Attacking the Lung

Common Pathogenesis	
Wind heat attacking the lung	
Manifestations	**Systematic Pathogenesis**
Cough	Dysfunction of the lung in dispersing and precipitating qi
Sticky, scant, and yellow sputum	Heat causing the body fluids to become concentrated
Yellow sticky nasal discharge, sore throat	Obstruction at the opening of the lung
Fever, chills, thin yellow tongue coating, and rapid floating pulse	Wind heat remaining in the exterior of the body

Main manifestations: Cough with yellow sticky sputum, combined with manifestations as seen in **exterior heat patterns (Table 6.7).**

Wind Cold Attacking the Lung

This pattern is caused by wind cold attacking the lung leading to a dysfunction of the lung in dispersing and precipitating (see Table 9.5).

Table 9.5 Wind Cold Attacking the Lung

Common Pathogenesis	
Wind cold attacking the lung	
Manifestations	**Systematic Pathogenesis**
Cough	Dysfunction of the lung in dispersing and precipitating qi
Clear thin white sputum	Body fluids producing phlegm when coming together
Runny nose with thin, clear discharge	Obstruction at opening of the lung
Chills and fever, headache, thin white tongue coating, tense floating pulse	Wind cold remaining in the exterior of the body

Main manifestations: Cough with thin white sputum, combined with manifestations as seen in **exterior cold patterns (Table 6.6).**

Dryness Attacking the Lung

This pattern is caused by dryness attacking the lung leading to an impairment of lung yin. It is also called exterior dryness pattern.

Table 9.6 Dryness Attacking the Lung

Common Pathogenesis	
Dryness attacking the lung	
Manifestations	**Systematic Pathogenesis**
Dry cough with sticky and scant sputum	Dysfunction of the lung in dispersing and precipitating qi
Pain in the chest, nasal bleeding, coughing blood	Impairment of the blood vessels in the lung
Dry throat, nose	Poor nourishment of the opening of the lung
Fever, chills, yellow thin tongue coating, rapid floating pulse	Dryness remaining in the exterior of the body

Main manifestations: Dry cough and sore throat, combined with manifestations as seen in **exterior dryness patterns (Table 7.5).**

Excess Heat Accumulating in the Lung

This pattern is brought about by excess heat accumulating in the lung, leading to a dysfunction of the lung in dispersing and precipitating qi.

Table 9.7 Excess Heat Accumulating in the Lung

Common Pathogenesis	
Excess heat accumulating in the lung	
Manifestations	**Systematic Pathogenesis**
Cough, asthma	Dysfunction of the lung in dispersing and precipitating qi
Pain in the chest	Impairment of the lung collateral channels leading to poor circulation of qi and blood
Sticky yellow sputum	Excess heat solidifying body fluids into phlegm

Expectoration of pus and blood	Excess heat putrefying flesh into pus
High fever, thirst, dry stools, dark colored urine	Excess heat impairing body fluids
Red tongue with yellow coating, rapid pulse with forceful beat	Excess heat spreading all over the body

Main manifestations: Cough, asthma with yellow sticky sputum, and chest pain, combined with manifestations as seen in **excess heat patterns (Table 6.9).**

Excess Cold Attacking the Lung

This pattern is caused by excess cold attacking the lung leading to a dysfunction of the lung in dispersing and precipitating.

Table 9.8 Excess Cold Attacking the Lung

Common Pathogenesis	
Excess cold attacking the lung	
Manifestations	**Systematic Pathogenesis**
Cough, asthma	Dysfunction of the lung in dispersing and precipitating qi
Thin white sputum	Phlegm fluids remaining in the lung
Aversion to cold, cold limbs	Yang qi failing to go out and warm the surface of the body, caused by stagnated phlegm inside the body
White tongue coating, deep tense pulse	Excess cold accumulating in the body

Main manifestations: Cough and asthma with white sputum, combined with manifestations as seen in **excess cold patterns (Table 6.12).**

Damp Phlegm Obstructing the Lung

This pattern is caused by damp phlegm obstructing the lung leading to a dysfunction of the lung in dispersing and precipitating.

Table 9.9 Damp Phlegm Obstructing the Lung

Common Pathogenesis	
Damp phlegm obstructing the lung	
Manifestations	**Systematic Pathogenesis**
Cough, asthma	Dysfunction of the lung in dispersing and precipitating qi
Copious sputum which is easy to expectorate	Phlegm stagnating in the lung
Fullness and oppression in the chest	Stagnation of lung qi
White greasy tongue coating, rolling pulse	Phlegm accumulation

Main manifestations: Cough, asthma with copious sputum, and fullness and oppression in the chest combined with manifestation as seen in **phlegm patterns (Table 7.9).**

Wind Water Attacking the Lung

This pattern is caused by pathogenic wind attacking the lung leading to a dysfunction of the lung in draining the water passage, with water damp penetrating the muscular interstices and skin.

Table 9.10 Wind Water Attacking the Lung

Common Pathogenesis	
Dysfunction of the lung in regulating water passage	
Manifestations	**Systematic Pathogenesis**
Sudden edema starting from the eyelids then spreading throughout the trunk and the limbs	Water retained in the muscular interstices and skin
Puffy face	Wind rising against water in the upper body
Oliguria	Dysfunction of the lung in draining water downwards to the bladder
Chills, fever, thin white tongue coating, and floating pulse	Wind remaining the exterior of the body

Main manifestations: Sudden occurrence of edema which starts with the eyelids then spreads to the trunk, and oliguria combined with manifestations as seen in **exterior cold patterns (Table 6.6)** and **water qi patterns (Table 7.11).**

3. DIFFERENTIAL DIAGNOSIS OF LUNG PATTERNS

It is often difficult to distinguish between patterns of dryness attacking the lung and lung yin deficiency as they both manifest with dry cough, as shown in Table 9.11. It is also difficult to distinguish between patterns of wind cold, excess cold attacking the lung, and damp phlegm obstructing the lung patterns, as they all present with cough and thin clear sputum. Therefore, a differential diagnosis is essential to determine the appropriate pattern, as shown in Table 9.12.

Table 9.11 Comparison Between Dryness Attacking the Lung and Lung Yin Deficiency

Pattern	Dryness attacking the lung	Deficiency of lung yin
Pathogenesis	Dryness attacking the lung leading to the impairment of lung yin	Lung yin deficiency leading to the rising of deficiency fire
Pattern Type	Exterior excess	Interior deficiency
Seasonal Tendency	Most prevalent in autumn	Possible in all seasons
Illness Duration	Short	Long
Common Manifestations	Cough, slight asthma, scant and sticky sputum with difficult expectoration	
Differentiating Manifestations	Fever, chills, dry nose and mouth with thirst, red tongue with thin coating, floating rapid pulse	Tidal fever, malar flush, night sweats, five-palm heat, red tongue with scant coating, thin rapid pulse

Table 9.12 Comparison Between Wind Cold Attacking the Lung, Excess Cold Attacking the Lung, and Damp Phlegm Obstructing the Lung

Pattern	Wind cold attacking the lung	Excess cold attacking the lung	Damp phlegm obstructing the lung
Syndrome Types	Exterior cold	Interior cold	Combined damp and phlegm
Common Manifestations	Cough with clear thin sputum, white tongue coating		
Differentiating Manifestations	Chills, slight fever, headache, stiff neck, lack of sweating	Aversion to cold, cold limbs with preference for warmth, no fever	Copious sputum that is easily expectorated
Tongue Condition	Thin white	White	White greasy
Pulse Condition	Floating and tense	Deep and tense	Rolling

II. Pattern Identification According to the Large Intestine

Pattern identification for disorders of the large intestine is based on understanding the physiological functions and pathological characteristics of the large intestine. The manifestations obtained from the four diagnostic methods are analyzed in this light and a final pattern diagnosis is achieved.

Large intestine disorders mainly involve the functions of the large intestine in transmission, and thus manifest as changes in stool and as abnormal sensations in the abdomen.

1. Main Analysis of Disorders of the Large Intestine

An analysis of the general manifestations and the pathogenesis for disorders of the large intestine is shown in Table 9.13.

Table 9.13 Analysis of Manifestations and Pathogenesis for the Large Intestine

Common Pathogenesis	
Dysfunction of the large intestine in transmission of food and waste	
Manifestations	**Systematic Pathogenesis**
Abdominal pain with cold sensation	Deficiency cold accumulating in the large intestine leading to poor warmth of the abdomen
Abdominal pain and distension	Stagnation of large intestine qi
Loose stools (to the point of dawn diarrhea) or collapse of the bowels	Kidney yang deficiency leading to failure of the life gate fire in generating earth (spleen)
Constipation	Excess heat damaging the body fluids, or a constitutional insufficiency of body fluids leading to poor lubrication of the intestinal tract
Bloody and purulent stools	Damp heat accumulating in the intestinal tract and impairing the blood vessels of the large intestine

2. Common Pattern Types

Pattern identification for disorders of the large intestine is based on understanding the physiological functions and pathological characteristics of the large intestine, in order to analyze manifestations obtained from four diagnostic methods and gain the final pattern diagnosis.

Disorders of the large intestine are affected by the lung because they are linked in an exterior-interior relationship.

Large intestine disorders commonly involve the functions of the large intestine in transmission, and thus manifest as changes in stools and abnormal sensations of the abdomen.

Damp Heat Accumulating in the Large Intestine

This pattern is caused by summerheat combined with damp attacking the large intestine or by the intake of improper or unclean food, leading to the dysfunction of the large intestine in transmission of food and waste.

Table 9.14 Damp Heat Accumulating in the Large Intestine

Common Pathogenesis	
Damp heat accumulating in the large intestine	
Manifestations	**Systematic Pathogenesis**
Abdominal pain, tenesmus	Qi stagnation in intestinal tract
Bloody and purulent stools	Impairment of the blood vessels leading to putrefying pustulating flesh
Loose stools with discomfort or burning sensation of the anus	Downward flow of damp heat
Thirst without desire to drink	Dysfunction of body fluids distribution
Yellow greasy tongue coating, soggy rapid pulse	Damp heat accumulating in the body

Main manifestations: Abdominal pain, abnormal defecation, yellow greasy tongue coating and rapid pulse, combined with manifestations as seen in **damp patterns (Table 7.4).**

Large Intestine Deficiency Cold

Large intestine deficiency cold pattern commonly results from chronic damage to the large intestine during a long-lasting illness.

Table 9.15 Large Intestine Deficiency Cold

Common Pathogenesis	
Yang qi deficiency in the large intestine	
Manifestations	**Systematic Pathogenesis**
Chronic diarrhea	Poor consolidation of the large intestine
Dull abdominal pain, preference for warmth and pressure	Poor warmth of the large intestine
Aversion to cold, cold limbs	Poor warmth of the body and limbs
White tongue coating, deep slow pulse with forceless beat	Deficiency cold accumulating inside the body

Main manifestations*:* Abdominal pain and diarrhea, combined with manifestations as seen in **yang deficiency patterns (Table 6.11).**

Large Intestine Yin (Fluids) Deficiency

Large intestine yin fluids deficiency often occurs in the elderly, in women after child-birth, or in the weak after a long-lasting illness.

Table 9.16 Large Intestine Yin (Fluids) Deficiency

Common Pathogenesis	
Yin (fluids) deficiency in the large intestine	
Manifestations	**Systematic Pathogenesis**
Dry stools, difficult defecation	Poor lubrication of the intestinal tract and weak promotion of the bowels
Thirst, dry mouth and tongue coating	Poor moistening of the mouth and tongue
Red tongue with scant and dry coating, thin and choppy pulse	Production of deficiency heat

Main manifestations: Dry stools and difficult defecation, combined with manifestations as seen in **yin deficiency patterns (Table 6.10).**

III. PATTERN IDENTIFICATION ACCORDING TO THE SPLEEN

The method of pattern identification for disorders of the spleen is based on understanding the physiological functions and pathological characteristics of the spleen. The manifestations obtained from the four diagnostic methods are analyzed in this light and a final pattern diagnosis is achieved.

Spleen disorders generally manifest as a dysfunction of the spleen in transformation and transportation.

1. MAIN ANALYSIS OF DISORDERS OF THE SPLEEN

Most patterns of spleen disorders are characterized by deficiency and involve damp. An analysis of the general manifestations and the pathogenesis for disorders of the spleen is shown in Table 9.17.

Table 9.17 Manifestations and Pathogenesis for Disorders of the Spleen

Common Pathogenesis	
Dysfunction of the spleen in transportation and transformation	
Manifestations	**Systematic Pathogenesis**
Sallow complexion, emaciation	Poor source of nutritive substances leading to poor nourishment of the limbs and body
Abdominal distension, poor appetite	Spleen qi stagnating in the middle burner leading to poor digestion
Loose stools	Downward flow of undigested substances to the large intestine
Edema	Dysfunction of the spleen in transporting damp, leading to the retention of body fluids
Bleeding	Dysfunction of the spleen in keeping blood circulating inside the blood vessels

2. COMMON PATTERN TYPES

Common patterns of spleen disorders are classified as either deficiency or excess patterns. The former are due to malnutrition, overexertion and emotional distress, or to poor nursing after a severe and chronic illness; the latter are caused by improper food intake, an attack of damp heat or cold damp, or inappropriate treatment.

Spleen Qi Deficiency

Spleen qi deficiency refers to a condition in which the spleen fails to carry out its function of transformation and transportation.

Table 9.18 Spleen Qi Deficiency

Common Pathogenesis	
Spleen qi deficiency	
Manifestations	**Systematic Pathogenesis**
Poor appetite, abdominal distension, loose stools	Dysfunction of the spleen in transportation and transformation
Listlessness, lassitude, low voice	Poor invigoration of the physical body and the vitality
Sallow complexion, pale tongue	Poor transformation of qi and blood
Weak pulse	Poor promotion of circulation in the blood vessels

Diagnosis in Traditional Chinese Medicine

Main manifestations: Poor appetite, abdominal distension, and loose stools, combined with manifestations as seen in **qi deficiency patterns (Table 8.2).**

Spleen Qi Fall

Spleen qi fall refers to a condition in which a spleen qi deficiency is marked by prolapse of internal organs.

Table 9.19 Spleen Qi Fall

Common Pathogenesis	
Spleen qi deficiency	
Manifestations	**Systematic Pathogenesis**
Poor appetite, abdominal distension with downbearing sensation, chronic loose stools	Dysfunction of the spleen in transportation and transformation
Listlessness, lassitude, low voice, emaciation	Poor invigoration of the physical body and the vitality
Sallow complexion, pale tongue, weak pulse	Poor transformation of qi and blood
Prolapse of internal organs such as rectum, uterus, stomach, or kidneys	Poor promotion of lucid yang qi leading to a poor hold on the internal organs

Main manifestations: Prolapse of internal organs combined with manifestations as seen in **spleen qi deficiency patterns (Table 9.18).**

Spleen Fails to Contain Blood inside the Vessels

This pattern is a condition in which spleen qi is insufficient, thus unable to keep blood circulating in the vessels.

Table 9.20 Spleen Fails to Contain Blood inside the Vessels

Common Pathogenesis	
Spleen qi deficiency	
Manifestations	**Systematic Pathogenesis**
All kinds of chronic bleeding such as bloody stools, bloody urine, and subcutaneous hemorrhage	Inability to govern blood circulating inside the blood vessels
Massive menstruation, menorrhalgia	Inability to consolidate the qi of the thoroughfare and controlling channels
Sallow, dry, or pale face	Poor nourishment of qi and blood

Poor appetite, abdominal distension, loose stools	Poor transportation by the spleen
Pale tongue	Poor production of blood and poor nourishment of tongue
Thin and weak pulse	Poor production of blood and poor filling of the vessels

Main manifestations: Bleeding combined with manifestations as seen in **spleen qi deficiency patterns (Table 9.18).**

Spleen Yang Deficiency

Spleen yang deficiency pattern refers to a condition in which spleen yang is insufficient, leading to poor warmth in the interior of the body.

Table 9.21 Spleen Yang Deficiency

Common Pathogenesis	
Spleen yang deficiency	
Manifestations	**Systematic Pathogenesis**
Poor appetite, abdominal distension, loose stools	Secondary to deficiency of spleen qi, leading to dysfunction of the spleen in transportation
Vague pain of the abdomen with preference for pressure and warmth	Poor warmth of the abdomen
Aversion to cold, cold limbs	Poor warmth of the body and limbs
No desire to drink	No impairment of the body fluids
Edema, scant urine	Body fluids retained in the skin
Leukorrhea with copious white vaginal discharge	Downward flow of cold damp
Pale and puffy tongue with tooth marks, white greasy tongue coating	Cold damp accumulating in the body
Deep and slow pulse with forceless beat	Poor promotion of qi circulating in the vessels

Main manifestations: Poor appetite, abdominal distension, and loose stools, combined with manifestations as seen in **yang deficiency patterns (Table 6.11).**

Cold Damp Accumulating in the Spleen

This refers to a condition in which cold damp accumulating in the spleen leads to problems in its ability to transform and transport.

Table 9.22 Cold Damp Accumulating in the Spleen

Common Pathogenesis	
Cold damp accumulating in the spleen	
Manifestations	**Systematic Pathogenesis**
Distension and fullness of the upper abdomen, poor appetite, loose stools	Dysfunction of the spleen in transportation and transformation
Nausea, vomiting	Reversal of stomach qi
Heaviness of the whole body and the head	Cold damp leading to obstructed qi and blood circulation
Edema, scant urine	Retention of body fluids
Leukorrhea with clear thin vaginal discharge	Downward flow of cold damp
Jaundice with dim yellow skin and whites of the eyes	Inability to soothe liver and gallbladder
White greasy tongue coating	Upward steaming of turbid damp
Soggy and slow pulse	Massive damp retained in the body

Main manifestations: Yin type jaundice, edema, leukorrhea with clear thin vaginal discharge, white tongue coating, and slow pulse, combined with manifestations as seen in **damp patterns (Table 7.4).**

Damp Heat Accumulating in the Spleen

This refers to a condition in which damp heat accumulates in the middle burner leading to poor transformation and transportation.

Table 9.23 Damp Heat Accumulating in the Spleen

Common Pathogenesis	
Damp heat accumulating in the spleen	
Manifestations	**Systematic Pathogenesis**
Fullness and distension of the upper abdomen, poor appetite, nausea and vomiting	Dysfunction of the spleen in transportation and transformation
Loose stools with discomfort in the anus, scant and dark urine, leukorrhea with yellow sticky vaginal discharge	Downward flow of damp heat

Bright yellow skin and whites of the eyes, itching	Damp heat steaming the gallbladder leading to an outflow of bile
Red tongue with yellow greasy coating, soggy rapid pulse	Damp heat retained in the body

Main manifestations: Yang type jaundice, leukorrhea with yellow sticky vaginal discharge, yellow tongue coating, and rapid pulse, combined with manifestations as seen in **damp patterns (Table 7.4).**

3. DIFFERENTIAL DIAGNOSIS OF DISORDERS OF THE SPLEEN

It is sometimes difficult to distinguish between the various patterns related to spleen qi deficiency and between conditions of damp heat versus cold damp disturbing the spleen. The two tables below provide information to differentiate these patterns.

Table 9.24 Comparison between Spleen Qi Deficiency, Spleen Qi Fall, and Failure of the Spleen to Keep Blood Circulating in the Vessels

Pattern	Spleen qi deficiency	Spleen qi fall	Spleen fails to contain blood inside the vessels
Common Pathogenesis	Spleen qi deficiency		
Systematic Pathogenesis	Dysfunction of the spleen in transportation and transformation	Dysfunction of the spleen in promoting lucid yang qi	Dysfunction of the spleen in keeping blood circulating in the vessels
Common Manifestations	Shortness of breath, lassitude, listlessness, low voice, no desire for speaking, spontaneous sweating; poor appetite, abdominal distension, loose stools; sallow complexion, pale tongue, and weak pulse		
Systematic Manifestations	Poor appetite, distension of the abdomen, loose stools	Prolapse of internal organs such as the rectum, stomach, uterus, kidneys	Bleeding in various locations, such as hemafecia, hematuria, subcutaneous hemorrhage

**Table 9.25 Comparison between Damp Heat and
Cold Damp Accumulating in the Spleen**

Pattern	Damp heat accumulating in the spleen	Cold damp accumulating in the spleen
Common Pathogenesis	Damp accumulating in the spleen leading to dysfunction in transportation and transformation	
Differentiating Pathogenesis	Combined with heat	Combined with cold
Common Manifestations	Sensation of fullness or oppression in the upper abdomen, heaviness of the head and the whole body, poor appetite, diarrhea, nausea, vomiting, greasy tongue coating, soft pulse	
Differentiating Manifestations	Feverish sensation of the body, dark colored urine, red tongue with yellow greasy coating, rapid soggy pulse	Cold sensation throughout the body, edema, scant urine, pale tongue with white greasy coating, slow soggy pulse

IV. PATTERN IDENTIFICATION ACCORDING TO THE STOMACH

The method of pattern identification for disorders of the stomach is based on understanding the physiological functions and pathological characteristics of the stomach. The manifestations obtained from the four diagnostic methods are analyzed in this light and a final pattern diagnosis is achieved.

Stomach disorders commonly involve the functions of the stomach in receiving food, transforming food into chyme, and sending digested food downwards. They manifest as changes in food intake, appetite, digestion, and sensations in the upper abdomen.

Stomach disorders are affected by the spleen because they are linked in an exterior-interior relationship.

1. MAIN ANALYSIS OF DISORDERS OF THE STOMACH

An analysis of the general manifestations and the pathogenesis for disorders of the stomach is shown in Table 9.26.

Table 9.26 Manifestations and Pathogenesis for Disorders of the Stomach

Common Pathogenesis	
Dysfunction of the stomach in storage and digestion	
Manifestations	**Systematic Pathogenesis**
Hyperactive appetite	Excess stomach fire leading to hyperfunction of the stomach
Abdominal pain with cold sensation	Excessive intake of raw cold food leading to restriction of stomach yang
Abdominal pain with hot sensation	Invasion of heat, excessive intake of greasy or hot food, leading to the production of stomach heat
Abdominal pain with abdominal distension	Food stagnation leading to stagnation of stomach qi
Dull pain of the gastric region	Deficiency cold of the stomach leading to poor warmth of the abdomen
Nausea, vomiting, belching, hiccups	Dysfunction of the stomach in precipitating qi, leading to reversal of stomach qi

2. COMMON PATTERN TYPES

Stomach disorders generally manifest as a dysfunction of the stomach in digestion. Common patterns are classified as either deficiency or excess patterns. The former are usually caused by irregular food intake, severe or chronic illness, or severe vomiting and diarrhea, causing the consumption of stomach qi, stomach yang, and stomach yin. The latter are often due to pathogenic cold or heat or improper food intake damaging the stomach.

Stomach Yin Deficiency

This refers to a condition in which stomach yin deficiency leads to poor lubrication of the stomach resulting in reversal of stomach qi.

Table 9.27 Stomach Yin Deficiency

Common Pathogenesis	
Deficiency of stomach yin	
Manifestations	**Systematic Pathogenesis**
Abdominal pain with burning sensation	Poor nourishment of the stomach in storing food and digesting
Hunger with no desire for food	Deficiency heat accumulating in the stomach leading to its inability to regulate stomach qi

Diagnosis in Traditional Chinese Medicine

Dry mouth and throat	Poor moistening of the mouth and throat
Nausea, hiccups	Reversal of stomach qi
Dry stools	Poor lubrication of the intestinal tract
Red tongue with scant coating and lack of saliva, thin rapid pulse	Deficiency fire flaring up and consuming body fluids

Main manifestations: Hunger without desire to eat, abdominal pain with burning sensation, combined with manifestations as seen in **yin deficiency patterns (Table 6.10)**, except for tidal fever, flushed zygomatic area, night sweats, and five-palm heat.

Stomach Deficiency Cold

This refers to a condition in which stomach yang deficiency leads to the production of deficiency cold resulting in reversal of stomach qi.

Table 9.28 Stomach Deficiency Cold

Common Pathogenesis	
Stomach yang deficiency	
Manifestations	**Systematic Pathogenesis**
Dull pain in the gastric region with preference for warmth and pressure	Poor warmth of the stomach
Poor appetite, distension and fullness of the upper abdomen	Dysfunction of the stomach in storage and digestion
Drooling with clear thin saliva	Inability to regulate the flow of stomach qi
No desire to drink, pale tongue with white coating, deep slow pulse with forceless beat	Deficiency cold accumulating in the body

Main manifestations: Poor appetite, fullness and distension of the upper abdomen, and drooling, combined with manifestations as seen in **yang deficiency patterns (Table 6.11).**

Excess Stomach Fire

This refers to a condition in which exuberant stomach fire leads to the failure of stomach qi to descend.

Table 9.29 Excess Stomach Fire

Common Pathogenesis	
Excess stomach fire	
Manifestations	**Systematic Pathogenesis**
Abdominal pain with burning sensation, swelling, bleeding, and pain of the teeth and gums, sores in the mouth	Flaring up of stomach fire leading to stagnation of qi and blood
Bad breath	Adverse upward steaming of turbid stomach qi
Hyperactive appetite	Hyperactivity of the stomach in storing food and digesting
Thirst with preference for cold drinks, constipation, dark scant urine	Impairment of body fluids
Red tongue with yellow coating, rapid pulse	Excess stomach heat accumulating in the body

Main manifestations: Abdominal pain with burning sensation, pain and swelling of the gums, parorexia and bad breath, combined with manifestations as seen in **excess heat patterns (Table 6.9).**

Cold Attacking the Stomach

This refers to pathogenic cold attacking the stomach leading to stomach qi failing to descend.

Table 9.30 Cold Attacking the Stomach

Common Pathogenesis	
Cold attacking the stomach	
Manifestations	**Systematic Pathogenesis**
Pain in the gastric region with cold sensation	Yang qi restrained in the interior of the body, failing to warm the upper abdomen
Severe pain occurring in the upper abdomen	Cold causing the blood vessels to contract, bringing about stagnation of qi and blood
Abdominal pain relieved by warmth	Warmth promoting yang qi
Drooling with clear saliva	Stagnation of qi from cold contraction leading to adverse upward flow of stomach qi
White tongue coating and deep tense pulse	Yang qi restricted by excess cold

Main manifestations: Painful abdomen with cold sensation, drooling, and deep tense pulse, combined with manifestations as seen in **excess cold patterns (Table 6.2).**

Food Stagnation

This refers to improper food intake leading to food being retained in the stomach.

Table 9.31 Food Stagnation

Common Pathogenesis	
Food stagnating in the stomach	
Manifestations	**Systematic Pathogenesis**
Overeating followed by distension, fullness, and pain of the gastric region	Undigested food retained in the stomach
Acid reflux, nausea, belching, and vomiting with foul smell	Reversal of stomach qi
Poor appetite	Impairment of stomach qi
Stools with foul smell	Downward flow of turbid qi
Thick greasy tongue coating	Upward steaming of turbid qi
Rolling pulse	Turbid damp accumulating in the body

Main manifestations: History of irregular food intake, abdominal distension and pain, belching, nausea, vomiting, and loose stools with foul smell, combined with manifestations as seen in **food stagnation patterns (Table 7.8).**

Blood Stasis in the Stomach

This refers to the condition of blood stasis in the stomach which is marked by a stabbing and fixed pain in the upper abdomen.

Table 9.32 Blood Stasis in the Stomach

Common Pathogenesis	
Blood stasis in the stomach	
Manifestations	**Systematic Pathogenesis**
Fixed stabbing pain in the gastric region	Obstruction of circulation of qi and blood
More severe abdominal pain after meals	Qi stagnation occurring after food intake
Hematochezia	Extravasation of blood
Purple tongue and choppy pulse	Obstruction of blood circulation

Main manifestations: Stabbing pain in the abdomen and stool containing blood, combined with manifestations as seen in **blood stasis patterns (Table 8.7).**

V. Pattern Identification According to the Heart

The method of pattern identification for disorders of the heart is based on understanding the physiological functions and pathological characteristics of the heart. The manifestations obtained from the four diagnostic methods are analyzed in this light and a final pattern diagnosis is achieved.

Heart disorders mainly involve the functions of the heart in governing blood circulation and consciousness.

1. Main Analysis of Disorders of the Heart

The common manifestations and pathogenesis for disorders of the heart are analyzed in Table 9.33.

Table 9.33 Manifestations and Pathogenesis for Disorders of the Heart

Manifestations	Common Pathogenesis	Systematic Pathogenesis
Pain in the cardiac region radiating to the shoulders and back	Dysfunction of the heart in governing blood circulation	Blockage of blood circulation
Palpitations		Insufficiency of heart qi, blood, yin, or yang leading to poor nourishment or invigoration of the heart
Insomnia		Flaring up of deficiency or excess heart fire; upward stirring of phlegm fire
Mental confusion or possibly loss of consciousness, delirium with high voice, irritability	Dysfunction of the heart in governing the mind leading to mental confusion and emotional changes	Upward stirring of phlegm fire
Loss of consciousness or drowsiness, dull reactions, low voice, shortness of breath		Insufficiency of heart qi
Emotional depression, muttering to oneself, dull expression, and preference for solitude		Accumulation of turbid phlegm
Emotional excitement, madness, shouting in a high voice, damaging furniture, offensive behavior		Upward flaring of phlegm fire affecting the mind
Red tongue tip, mouth ulcers	Tongue is the external appearance of the heart	Flaring up of heart fire

2. COMMON PATTERN TYPES

Common patterns of the heart are classified into two groups. Deficiency patterns are caused by congenital defects, overanxiety, weak ancestral qi, or chronic illness, leading to a deficiency of heart qi, heart yang, heart blood, and heart yin. Excess patterns are mainly caused by phlegm, fire, cold, qi stagnation, and blood stasis.

Heart Qi Deficiency

Heart qi deficiency pattern refers to a condition in which insufficient heart qi leads to a poor promotion of heart blood.

Table 9.34 Heart Qi Deficiency

Common Pathogenesis	
Insufficiency of heart qi	
Manifestations	**Systematic Pathogenesis**
Palpitations, dizziness, weak pulse	Poor promotion of blood circulation
Oppression of the chest, shortness of breath	Poor promotion of qi flow in the chest
Lassitude, listlessness	Poor invigoration of the physical body and the vitality
Spontaneous sweating	Poor consolidation of the surface of the body
All manifestations aggravated by exercise	Exercise consuming qi
Pale face and tongue	Poor nourishment of the face and the tongue
Knotted or intermittent pulse	Poor promotion of blood circulation

Main manifestations: Palpitations and oppression of the chest, combined with manifestations as seen in **qi deficiency patterns (Table 8.2).**

Heart Yang Deficiency

Heart yang deficiency pattern refers to a condition in which insufficient heart yang leads to deficiency cold, resulting in poor warmth of the body and poor promotion of blood circulation.

Table 9.35 Heart Yang Deficiency

Common Pathogenesis	
Insufficiency of heart yang	
Manifestations	**Systematic Pathogenesis**
Occasional attacks of colic pain in the cardiac region, oppression of the chest	Poor warmth of qi and blood leading to an obstruction in their circulation
Aversion to cold, cold limbs	Poor warmth of the whole body and limbs
Pale tongue with tooth marks	Poor transportation and transformation of body fluids
Knotted or intermittent pulse	Poor promotion of blood circulation

Main manifestations: Occasional pain in the cardiac region, combined with manifestations as seen in **yang deficiency patterns (Table 6.11)**.

Sudden Collapse of Heart Yang

Sudden collapse of heart yang pattern refers to a severe condition in which a sudden collapse of heart yang leads to poor warmth of the body and poor promotion of blood circulation. Note that clinically "heart attack" is diagnosed as heart yang collapse.

Table 9.36 Sudden Collapse of Heart Yang

Common Pathogenesis	
Sudden collapse of heart yang	
Manifestations	**Systematic Pathogenesis**
Palpitations, sudden attacks of cardiac pain	Failure to promote blood circulation
Face suddenly turning pale, purple lips and tongue	Obstruction of heart blood
Profuse cold sweat, cold limbs, weak breathing	Collapse of yang qi leading to poor warmth of the whole body and limbs
Indistinct pulse	Inability to promote blood circulation

Main manifestations: Palpitations, sudden attacks of cardiac pain, combined with manifestations as seen in **yang exhaustion patterns (Table 6.29)**.

Heart Blood Deficiency

Heart blood deficiency pattern refers to a condition in which there is insufficient heart blood to nourish the heart and mind.

Table 9.37 Heart Blood Deficiency

Common Pathogenesis	
Insufficiency of heart blood	
Manifestations	**Systematic Pathogenesis**
Palpitations, forgetfulness, poor concentration	Poor nourishment of the heart
Insomnia	Poor nourishment of the mind leading to instability of vital qi
Dizziness, pale face	Poor upward nourishment of the head and face
Thin pulse	Poor filling of the blood vessels

Main manifestations: Palpitations, forgetfulness, poor concentration, and insomnia, combined with manifestations as seen in **blood deficiency patterns (Table 8.6).**

Heart Yin Deficiency

Heart yin deficiency pattern refers to a condition in which insufficient heart yin leads to the production of deficiency fire.

Table 9.38 Heart Yin Deficiency

Common Pathogenesis	
Insufficiency of heart yin	
Manifestations	**Systematic Pathogenesis**
Palpitations, insomnia, dream-disturbed sleep	Poor nourishment of the heart and mind
Tidal fever, malar flush, five-palm heat, irritability	Upward stirring of deficiency fire affecting the mind
Night sweats	Deficiency fire compressing body fluids outward
Red tongue with scant coating, thin rapid pulse	Deficiency fire spreading all over the body

Main manifestations: Palpitations, insomnia, and dream-disturbed sleep, combined with manifestations as seen in **yin deficiency patterns (Table 6.10).**

Upward Flaring of Heart Fire

Upward flaring of heart fire refers to a condition of exuberant heart fire stirring upwards.

Table 9.39 Upward Flaring of Heart Fire

Common Pathogenesis	
Flaring up of heart fire	
Manifestations	**Systematic Pathogenesis**
Palpitations, irritability, insomnia	Restlessness of the mind
Red tongue tip, sores of the mouth and the tongue	The tongue is the sprout of the heart
Thirst, dark urine, constipation	Impairment of body fluids
Red tongue with yellow coating and rapid pulse	Excess fire accumulating in the body

Main manifestations: Palpitations, insomnia, red tongue ti,p and sores of the mouth and the tongue, combined with manifestations as seen in **excess heat patterns (Table 6.9).**

Obstruction of the Heart Vessel

Obstruction of the heart vessel pattern can be due to blood stasis, qi stagnation, phlegm accumulation, or cold accumulation. These are shown in the tables below.

Table 9.40 Obstruction of Heart Vessel due to Blood Stasis

Common Pathogenesis	
Heart blood not circulating smoothly in the heart vessel	
Manifestations	**Systematic Pathogenesis**
Palpitations	Poor nourishment of the heart
Stabbing pain in the cardiac region radiating to the back and the medial side of the arms, purple tongue	Blockage of blood circulation
Wiry choppy pulse	Dysfunction of the liver in regulating qi flow

Main manifestations: Palpitations; stabbing pain in the cardiac region radiating to the back, shoulders, and medial side of the arms, combined with manifestations as seen in **blood stasis patterns (Table 8.7).**

Table 9.41 Obstruction of Heart Vessel Due to Qi Stagnation

Common Pathogenesis	
Stagnation of qi flow	
Manifestations	**Systematic Pathogenesis**
Palpitations	Irregular flow of heart qi
Distending pain in the cardiac region radiating to the back and the medial side of the arms; aggravated by mental depression	Blockage of blood circulation
Wiry choppy pulse	Dysfunction of the liver in regulating qi flow

Main manifestations: Palpitations, distending pain in the cardiac region radiating to the back, shoulders, and the medial side of the arms, combined with manifestations as seen in **qi stagnation patterns (Table 8.4).**

Table 9.42 Obstruction of Heart Vessel due to Phlegm Accumulation

Common Pathogenesis	
Phlegm accumulating in the heart vessel	
Manifestations	**Systematic Pathogenesis**
Palpitations	Poor circulation of heart blood leading to poor nourishment of the heart
Sensation of choking pain and oppression in the cardiac region, radiating to the back and the medial side of the arms	Obstruction of blood circulation
Thick greasy tongue coating and rolling pulse	Turbid phlegm accumulating in the body and steaming outward

Main manifestations: Palpitations, pain in the cardiac region radiating to the back, shoulders, and the medial side of the arms, combined with manifestations as seen in **phlegm patterns (Table 7.9).**

Table 9.43 Obstruction of Heart Vessel Due to Accumulation of Cold

Common Pathogenesis	
Excess cold contracting the blood vessels	
Manifestations	**Systematic Pathogenesis**
Palpitations	Obstruction of blood circulation

Pain in the cardiac region relieved by warmth, deep slow pulse	Warmth promoting blood circulation
Aversion to cold, cold limbs	Poor warmth of the body

Main manifestations: Palpitations, pain in the cardiac region radiating to the back, shoulders, and the medial side of the arms, combined with manifestations as seen in **excess cold patterns (Table 6.12).**

Upward Flaring of Phlegm Fire Affecting the Mind

This refers to phlegm fire flaring upward leading to restlessness of the mind.

Table 9.44 Upward Flaring of Phlegm Fire Affecting the Mind

Common Pathogenesis	
Phlegm fire flaring upward	
Manifestations	**Systematic Pathogenesis**
Mania, agitation, anxiety, easily-arising anger, incessant talking, ranting and raving, crying and laughing, offensive behavior	Upward flaring of phlegm fire affecting the mind
Palpitations, irritability, insomnia	Unsteadiness of the mind
Thirst	Impairment of yin fluids
Yellow greasy tongue coating, rolling and rapid pulse	Phlegm fire accumulating in the body

Main manifestations: Mania, madness, irritability, and thirst, combined with manifestations as seen in **phlegm patterns (Table 7.9).**

Phlegm Misting the Mind

This refers to a condition of stirring of turbid phlegm affecting the mind and leading to mental confusion. There are three variations of this pattern as shown in Table 9.45.

Table 9.45 Phlegm Misting the Mind

Pattern types	Manifestations	Systematic Pathogenesis
Severe cases of any disease	Fuzzy thoughts, mental confusion, possibly loss of consciousness, wheezing in the throat	Accumulation of phlegm caused by qi stagnation leading to dysfunction of the heart in governing the mind

Depressive psychosis	Depression, introversion, apathy, muttering, dull reactions, dull-looking expression	Dysfunction of the heart in governing vitality
Epilepsy with seizures	Sudden loss of consciousness, stiff limbs, convulsions of the extremities, drooling with foamy saliva, wheezing sound in the throat	Accumulation of wind phlegm in the heart affecting the mind

Main manifestations: Mental confusion and loss of consciousness, combined with manifestations as seen in **phlegm patterns (Table 7.9).**

3. DIFFERENTIAL DIAGNOSIS OF DISORDERS OF THE HEART

It is sometimes difficult to distinguish between deficiency of heart qi, heart yang, heart blood, heart yin, and sudden collapse of heart yang, so the differential diagnoses for these are shown in Table 9.46. There are also different subcategories under obstruction of the heart vessel patterns which are shown in Table 9.47.

Table 9.46 Comparison of Deficiency Patterns of the Heart

Common Manifestations		
Palpitations		
Patterns	**Differentiating Manifestations**	**Systematic Pathogenesis**
Heart qi deficiency	Oppression of the chest, shortness of breath, spontaneous sweating	Insufficiency of heart qi
Heart yang deficiency	Occasional pain in the cardiac region, cold limbs, puffy face and tongue, edema	Insufficiency of heart yang
Heart yang collapse	Sudden attacks of pain in the cardiac region, cold sweats, sudden paleness of the face	Sudden collapse of heart yang
Heart vessel obstruction	Pain in the cardiac region radiating to the back and the medial side of the forearms, purple tongue, choppy pulse	Obstructed blood circulation
Heart blood deficiency	Insomnia, forgetfulness, poor concentration	Insufficiency of heart blood
Heart yin deficiency	Insomnia, irritability, five-palm heat, night sweats	Insufficiency of heart yin

Table 9.47 Comparison of Types of Obstruction of the Heart Vessel

Common Manifestations		
Palpitations, cardiac pain radiating to the shoulders, the back, and the medial side of the arms; uneven pulse, purple tongue		
Patterns	**Differentiating Manifestations**	**Systematic Pathogenesis**
Blood stasis	Stabbing pain fixed in the cardiac region, purple tongue	Stagnated blood circulation
Qi stagnation	Distending pain in the cardiac region, affected by emotional changes	Qi stagnation leading to blood stasis
Phlegm accumulation	Sensation of choking pain and oppression in the cardiac region, obesity, greasy tongue coating, rolling pulse	Phlegm accumulation leading to blood stasis
Qi deficiency	Dull pain with oppression of the chest, shortness of breath, spontaneous sweating, pale purple tongue, weak pulse	Qi deficiency leading to poor promotion of blood circulation
Cold accumulation	Pain in the cardiac region relieved by warmth, aversion to cold, cold limbs, white tongue coating, deep slow pulse	Excess cold contracting the blood vessels, leading to stagnated blood circulation

VI. PATTERN IDENTIFICATION ACCORDING TO THE SMALL INTESTINE

The method of pattern identification for disorders of the small intestine is based on understanding the physiological functions and pathological characteristics of the small intestine. The manifestations obtained from the four diagnostic methods are analyzed in this light and a final pattern diagnosis is achieved.

Disorders of the small intestine commonly involve the functions of the small intestine in storing and digesting food, and in lifting up lucid nutrition and sending down turbid wastes. Therefore, they manifest as changes in digestion, defecation, and urination, and in sensations in the abdomen.

Small intestine disorders are involved with heart disorders because they are linked in an exterior-interior relationship.

1. MAIN ANALYSIS OF DISORDERS OF THE SMALL INTESTINE

An analysis of the general manifestations and the pathogenesis for disorders of the small intestine is shown in Table 9.48.

Table 9.48 Manifestations and Pathogenesis of Small Intestine Disorders

Common Pathogenesis	
Dysfunction of the small intestine in storing and digesting, and in separating lucid nutrition from turbid waste	
Manifestations	**Systematic Pathogenesis**
Loose stools	Failure of the small intestine to separate food and waste
Abdominal pain	Deficiency cold accumulating in the small intestine leading to poor warmth of the abdomen; or qi stagnating in the small intestine leading to an obstruction of latent qi
Dark scant urine, hot sensation of urethral tract	Downward flow of damp heat
Hematuria	Excess heat accumulating in the small intestine, moving down to the bladder and impairing the blood vessels

2. COMMON PATTERN TYPES

Common patterns of the small intestine are classified into small intestine deficiency cold, excess heat or excess cold accumulating in the small intestine, and small intestine qi obstruction.

Small Intestine Deficiency Cold

This refers to a condition of cold from yang deficiency accumulating in the lower abdomen.

Table 9.49 Small Intestine Deficiency Cold

Common Pathogenesis	
Insufficiency of small intestine yang	
Manifestations	**Systematic Pathogenesis**
Dull pain in the lower abdomen with preference for warmth and pressure	Poor warmth of the abdomen
Borborygmus, loose stools retaining undigested food	Downward flow of undigested food to the large intestine
Scant and clear urine	Massive amounts of body fluids excreted from the large intestine with stools
Pale tongue with white coating, deep slow pulse	Deficiency cold accumulating in the body

Main manifestations: Abdominal pain and loose stools containing undigested food, combined with manifestations as seen in **yang deficiency patterns (Table 6.11).**

Small Intestine Excess Heat

This refers to a condition of excess heat accumulating in the lower abdomen.

Table 9.50 Small Intestine Excess Heat

Common Pathogenesis	
Excess heat accumulating in the small intestine	
Manifestations	**Systematic Pathogenesis**
Painful urination with burning sensation in the opening of the urethral tract	Heart fire moving down to the small intestine
Scant dark urine	Excess heat consuming body fluids
Irritability, sores in tongue and mouth	Upward stirring of heart fire affecting the mind
Red tongue with yellow coating, rapid pulse	Excess fire accumulating in the body

Main manifestations: Painful urination with burning sensation and sores in the mouth and on the tongue, combined with manifestations as seen in **excess heat patterns (Table 6.9).**

Small Intestine Qi Obstruction

This refers to a severe condition in which material pathogens are obstructing the intestinal tract, leading to qi stagnation and blood stasis.

Table 9.51 Small Intestine Qi Obstruction

Common Pathogenesis	
Qi obstructing the small intestine	
Manifestations	**Systematic Pathogenesis**
Colic and paroxysmal pain in the abdomen	Obstruction of small intestine qi
Progressive abdominal distension	Blockage of latent qi
Vomiting	Reversal of stomach qi
Constipation without flatus from the bowels	Dysfunction of the small intestine in transportation

Main manifestations: Paroxysmal abdominal pain and progressive abdominal distension, combined with manifestations as seen in **qi stagnation patterns (Table 8.4).**

Small Intestine Cold Accumulation

This refers to a condition of excess cold accumulating the lower abdomen.

Table 9.52 Small Intestine Cold Accumulation

Common Pathogenesis	
Cold accumulation leading to qi stagnation in the small intestine	
Manifestations	**Systematic Pathogenesis**
Severe pain in the abdomen radiating upward to the lumbar region and back, and downward to the testes	Stagnation of small intestine qi
Hernia marked by swelling and downbearing pain radiating down to the scrotum	Qi stagnation leading to blood stasis
White tongue coating, deep tense pulse	Excess cold accumulating in the body

Main manifestations: Spasmodic pain in the lower abdomen radiating to the testes and swollen testes, combined with manifestations as seen in **excess cold patterns (Table 6.12).**

VII. PATTERN IDENTIFICATION ACCORDING TO THE LIVER

The method of pattern identification for disorders of the liver is based on understanding the physiological functions and pathological characteristics of the liver. The manifestations obtained from the four diagnostic methods are analyzed in this light and a final pattern diagnosis is achieved.

Liver disorders mainly involve the functions of the liver in dispersing and precipitating, and thus manifest as emotional depression, irritability, distending pain, and convulsions and trembling of the limbs and the body.

1. MAIN ANALYSIS OF DISORDERS OF THE LIVER

The common manifestations and pathogenesis for disorders of the liver are analyzed in Table 9.53.

Table 9.53 Manifestations and Pathogenesis for Disorders of the Liver

Common Pathogenesis	
Dysfunction of the liver in dispersing and precipitating	
Manifestations	**Systematic Pathogenesis**
Mental depression, sighing, irritability, distending pain in the chest, hypochondrium, breast, and lower abdomen, and wiry pulse	Liver qi stagnating in the chest, hypochondrium, and abdomen and stirring upward

Jaundice	Liver qi failing to soothe the gallbladder, leading to an outflow of bile
Dizziness, vertigo, convulsions of the limbs, trembling of the fingers and toes, and twitching of the muscles	Stirring up of liver wind

Common Pathogenesis	
Dysfunction of the liver in storing blood	
Manifestations	**Systematic Pathogenesis**
Blurred vision, floaters, color blindness, night blindness	Insufficiency of liver blood leading to poor nourishment of the eyes
Irregular menstruation including dysmenorrhea, amenorrhea, irregular menstrual cycle	Stagnation of liver qi leading to blood stasis; or constriction of the liver channel due to excess cold; or poor filling of thoroughfare and controlling channels due to liver blood deficiency

2. COMMON PATTERN TYPES

Common patterns of liver disorders are classified into two groups, excess and deficiency. Most of these patterns, though, are characterized by excess.

Liver Qi Stagnation

This refers to a condition of emotional depression leading to liver qi failing to spread freely and precipitate.

Table 9.54 Liver Qi Stagnation

Common Pathogenesis	
Liver qi stagnation	
Manifestations	**Systematic Pathogenesis**
Mental depression	Upward movement of phlegm from spleen mists the mind
Frequent sighing	Upward movement of reversed liver qi
Fullness, distending pain, or discomfort of the chest, hypochondrium, breasts, and lower abdomen; wiry pulse	Dysfunction of the liver in spreading and precipitating, leading to qi stagnating in the liver channel
Irregular menstruation, dysmenorrhea, amenorrhea	Dysfunction of the thoroughfare and controlling channels in regulating the menses
Poor appetite	Dysfunction of the spleen in transportation and

	transformation
Globus hystericus (plum-pit qi)	Phlegm combined with qi accumulating in the throat
Goiter	Phlegm combined with qi accumulating in the neck

Main manifestations: Mental depression, sighing, disorders of menstruation, plum-pit qi, and goiter, combined with manifestations as seen in **qi stagnation patterns (Table 8.4).**

Liver Blood Deficiency

This refers to a condition of insufficiency of liver blood leading to poor nourishment of the tissues and organs related to the liver.

Table 9.545 Liver Blood Deficiency

Common Pathogenesis	
Insufficiency of liver blood	
Manifestations	**Systematic Pathogenesis**
Pale face and tongue, dizziness, vertigo, tinnitus	Poor nourishment of the head
Numbness of the extremities and skin, tingling fingers or toes, sensation like crawling ants on skin, muscle twitching, pale, ridged, and/or brittle nails	Poor nourishment of the body
Blurred vision, floaters, night blindness, and color blindness	Poor nourishment of the opening of the liver
Delayed, short, scant menses light red in color, or amenorrhea	Poor filling of the thoroughfare and controlling channels

Main manifestations: Blurred vision, numbness of the body, and delayed and scant menstruation, combined with manifestations as seen in **blood deficiency patterns (Table 8.6).**

Liver Yin Deficiency

This refers to a condition of insufficient liver yin leading to the production of deficiency heat.

Table 9.56 Liver Yin Deficiency

Common Pathogenesis	
Insufficiency of liver yin	
Manifestations	**Systematic Pathogenesis**
Dizziness, tinnitus	Poor nourishment of the head
Blurred vision with dryness and discomfort of the eyes	Poor nourishment of the eyes (the opening of the liver)
Pain in the hypochondrium with burning sensation	Poor nourishment of the liver channel
Tidal fever, nocturnal fever, malar flush, night sweats, five-palm heat, red tongue with scant coating, wiry thin rapid pulse	Deficiency heat accumulating in the body

Main manifestations: Dizziness, tinnitus, and blurred vision with dryness and discomfort of the eyes and burning sensation of the hypochondrium, combined with manifestations as seen in **yin deficiency patterns (Table 6.10).**

Liver Fire Flaring Upward

This refers to a condition of liver fire flaring upward and steaming outward.

Table 9.57 Liver Fire Flaring Upward

Common Pathogenesis	
Liver fire accumulating in the body	
Manifestations	**Systematic Pathogenesis**
Flushed face, bloodshot eyes, dizziness, headache with distension, tinnitus, deafness, painful ears, irritability, red tongue with yellow coating, wiry rapid pulse	Liver fire stirring upward
Dry mouth, bitter taste in mouth	Gallbladder qi steaming upward
Dry stools and scant dark-colored urine	Excess fire impairing body fluids

Main manifestations: Distending pain of the head, dizziness, flushed face, bloodshot eyes, and irritability, combined with manifestations as seen in **excess heat patterns (Table 6.9).**

Liver Yang Rising

This refers to a condition of liver and kidney yin deficiency leading to liver yang rising.

Table 9.58 Liver Yang Rising

Common Pathogenesis	
Deficiency of liver and kidney yin in the lower body with liver yang rising in the upper body	
Manifestations	**Systematic Pathogenesis**
Headache with distension, dizziness, vertigo, tinnitus, flushed face, bloodshot eyes	Liver yang rising followed by upward stirring of qi and blood
Soreness and flaccidity of the lumbar region and knees	Poor nourishment of the lumbar region and the limbs
Heaviness of the head and possibly the upper body	Yang rising in the upper body
Irritability	Dysfunction of the liver in freely spreading and precipitating
Red tongue, wiry or wiry thin pulse	Deficiency heat accumulating in the body

Main manifestations: Distending pain of the head, dizziness, flushed face, bloodshot eyes, irritability, and heaviness of the head, combined with manifestations as seen in **yin deficiency patterns (Table 6.10).**

Liver Wind

Liver wind patterns can be due to liver yang rising, extreme heat, liver yin deficiency, or blood deficiency. These are shown in Tables 9.59 to 9.62.

Table 9.59 Liver Wind due to Liver Yang Rising

Common Pathogenesis	
Liver yang rising leading to an attack of liver wind	
Manifestations	**Systematic Pathogenesis**
Dizziness, vertigo, headache, irritability	Rising yang bring the qi and blood upward
Sudden onset of hemiparalysis, deviation of the eyes and mouth, drooling	Accumulation of wind phlegm in the channels and network vessels
Difficult speech	Wind phlegm obstructing the tongue vessel
Heaviness of the head and lightness of foot, soreness and weakness of lumbar area and knees, red tongue with scant coating, wiry thin pulse	Yin deficiency combined with yang hyperactivity

Main manifestations: Dizziness, vertigo, headache, and paralysis with difficult speech, combined with manifestations as seen in **liver yang rising patterns (Table 9.58).**

Table 9.60 Liver Wind due to Extreme Heat

Common Pathogenesis	
Extreme heat leading to an attack of liver wind	
Manifestations	**Systematic Pathogenesis**
High fever, flushed face, red eyes	Excess heat going outward
Convulsions of the body, opisthotonos	Extreme heat stirring up liver wind
Red tongue with yellow coating	Excess heat flaring up

Main manifestations: High fever, convulsions, and opisthotonos, combined with manifestations as seen in **excess heat patterns (Table 6.9).**

Table 9.61 Liver Wind due to Liver Yin Deficiency

Common Pathogenesis	
Liver yin deficiency leading to deficiency wind	
Manifestations	**Systematic Pathogenesis**
Dizziness, tinnitus	Poor nourishment of the head
Dryness and discomfort of the eyes, blurred vision	Poor nourishment of the opening of the liver
Involuntary extending or flexing motions, trembling of the fingers and toes	Poor nourishment of the tendons and muscles
Nocturnal fever, malar flush, five-palm heat, night sweats, red tongue, thin rapid pulse	Deficiency heat accumulating in the body

Main manifestations: Involuntary movement of the limbs, combined with manifestations as seen in **yin deficiency patterns (Table 6.10).**

Table 9.62 Liver Wind due to Liver Blood Deficiency

Common Pathogenesis	
Liver blood deficiency leading to deficiency wind	
Manifestations	**Systematic Pathogenesis**
Dizziness; pale face, lips, and tongue	Poor nourishment of the head

Blurred vision, floaters, or night blindness	Poor nourishment of the eyes
Numbness of the skin and limbs, tingling fingers and toes, pale and brittle nails	Poor nourishment of the body
Involuntary twitching of the muscles	Blood deficiency leading to poor nourishment
Wiry thin pulse	Poor filling of the blood vessels

Main manifestations: Tremors of the extremities and muscular twitching and cramping, combined with manifestations as seen in **blood deficiency patterns (Table 8.6).**

Liver Channel Damp Heat

This refers to a condition of damp heat accumulating in the liver and gallbladder channels leading to bile penetrating the skin. It presents as yang type jaundice.

Table 9.63 Liver Channel Damp Heat

Common Pathogenesis	
Damp heat accumulating in the liver channel	
Manifestations	**Systematic Pathogenesis**
Pain in the hypochondrium, distension and fullness of the upper abdomen, poor appetite, wiry rapid pulse	Dysfunction of the liver in dispersing and spreading freely
Jaundice marked by bright yellow color in the skin and the sclera	Damp heat steaming bile outward
Redness, blisters, shingles, eczema, skin lesions in the pudendal region; nocturnal emissions; swelling, pain, and distension with hot sensation of the scrotum; leukorrhea with yellow, thick, and sticky discharge; genital itching and genital herpes	Downward flow of damp heat along the liver channel
Bitter taste in mouth, red tongue with yellow greasy coating	Damp heat steaming gallbladder qi upwards
Pain in the hypochondrium, distension and fullness of the upper abdomen, poor appetite, wiry rapid pulse	Dysfunction of the liver in dispersing and spreading freely

Main manifestations: Jaundice, skin lesions in the pudendal region, and leukorrhagia, combined with manifestations as seen in **damp heat patterns (Table 7.4).**

Cold Accumulating in the Liver Channel

This refers to excess cold accumulating in the liver channel and causing pain.

Table 9.64 Cold Accumulating in the Liver Channel

Common Pathogenesis	
Excess cold accumulating in the liver channel	
Manifestations	**Systematic Pathogenesis**
Pain in the scrotum radiating to the lower abdomen with coldness, downbearing, and distending sensation in men, or pain in the lower abdomen radiating to the pudendal region with spasmodic sensation in women	Poor warmth and poor circulation of qi and blood
Aversion to cold, cold limbs	Yang qi restricted in the body, leading to inability to warm the body and limbs
Pale tongue with white coating, wiry tense pulse	Coldness tending to contract the blood vessels

Main manifestations: Pain with cold sensation in the pudendal region, combined with manifestations as seen in **excess cold patterns (Table 6.12).**

3. DIFFERENTIAL DIAGNOSIS OF DISORDERS OF THE LIVER

There are significant differences between conditions caused by liver fire flaring up versus hyperactive liver yang stirring upward and among the four subcategories of **liver wind patterns**, as shown in **Tables 9.65 and 9.66.**

Table 9.65 Comparison Between Liver Fire Flaring Upward and Liver Yang Rising

Pattern	Liver fire flaring upward	Liver yang rising
Pathogenesis	Excess fire accumulating in the liver channel	Kidney and liver yin weakening in the lower body with liver yang rising in the upper body
Pattern Type	Excess heat	Excess in the upper body with deficiency in the lower body
Illness Duration	Short	Long
Common Manifestations	Distending pain of the head, flushed face, bloodshot eyes, tinnitus, irritability	

	Fever, thirst, bitter taste in mouth, hypochondriac pain, dry stools, dark-colored urine, red tongue with yellow coating, wiry rapid pulse with forceful beat	Soreness and flaccidity of the lumbar region and knees, heaviness of the head, nights-weats, five palm heat, red tongue with scant coating, wiry thin rapid pulse
Differentiating Manifestations		

Table 9.66 Comparison Among Types of Liver Wind Patterns

Pattern	Liver yang rising	Extreme heat	Yin deficiency	Blood deficiency
Main Manifestations	Dizziness, vertigo, sudden hemiparaly-sis, deviation of the eyes and mouth	Convulsion of the extremities, opisthotonos	Involuntary convulsions of the extremities	Tremors of the muscles
Accompanying Manifestations	Dysphoria, malar flush, sore weak lumbar and knees	High fever, irritability, delirium, possi-bly loss of con-sciousness	Tidal fever, malar flush, night sweats, five-palm heat, sore weak lumbar and knees	Numbness and pain of the skin and knees; dizzi-ness; pale face, lips, and nails
Tongue Condition	Red tongue with greasy coating	Red tongue with yellow and dry coating	Red tongue with scant coating	Pale tongue with white coating
Pulse Condition	Wiry, thin, and rapid	Wiry and rapid with forceful beat	Wiry, thin, and rapid	Wiry and thin
Pathogenesis	Kidney and liver yin weakening the lower body with liver yang rising in the upper body	Excess heat accumulating in the body	Insufficiency of liver and kidney yin	Insufficiency of liver blood

VIII. PATTERN IDENTIFICATION ACCORDING TO THE GALLBLADDER

The method of pattern identification for disorders of the gallbladder is based on under-standing the physiological functions and pathological characteristics of the gallbladder. The manifestations obtained from the four diagnostic methods are analyzed in this light and a fi-nal pattern diagnosis is achieved.

Gallbladder disorders commonly involve the functions of the gallbladder in storing bile and helping the spleen and stomach to perform digestion, as well as affecting emotions. Thus, gallbladder disorders manifest as changes in the metabolism of bile, digestion, emotion, and sensations in the right hypochondrium. Disorders of the gallbladder are affected by the liver because they are closely linked in an exterior-interior relationship.

1. MAIN ANALYSIS OF DISORDERS OF THE GALLBLADDER

An analysis of the general manifestations and the pathogenesis for disorders of the gallbladder is shown in Table 9.67.

Table 9.67 Manifestations and Pathogenesis for Disorders of the Gallbladder

Common Pathogenesis	
Dysfunction of the gallbladder in dispersing and spreading	
Manifestations	**Systematic Pathogenesis**
Distension and pain in the hypochondrium	Stagnation of gallbladder qi
Jaundice, bitter taste in mouth	Steaming of gallbladder qi
Palpitations due to fright, insomnia, waking up in fright	Instability of gallbladder qi
Irritability, dizziness, tinnitus	Stirring up of gallbladder heat

2. COMMON PATTERN TYPES

There are only two common patterns of gallbladder disorders.

Gallbladder Depression-Phlegm Fire Stirring Upward

This refers to a condition of stagnation of gallbladder qi combined with phlegm fire stirring upward.

Table 9.68 Gallbladder Qi Stagnation-Phlegm Fire Stirring Upward

Common Pathogenesis	
Dysfunction of the gallbladder in dispersing and spreading, combined with phlegm fire stirring upward	
Manifestations	**Systematic Pathogenesis**
Insomnia, waking in fright, palpitations due to fright, irritability, wiry rapid pulse	Instability of gallbladder qi
Bitter taste in mouth, yellow greasy tongue coating	Steaming of gallbladder qi
Dizziness, tinnitus, irritability	Upward flaring of phlegm fire

Main manifestations: Palpitations due to fright, waking up in fright, insomnia, and bitter taste in the mouth, combined with manifestations as seen in **excess heat patterns (Table 6.9).**

Gallbladder Channel Damp Heat

This pattern refers to conditions of damp heat accumulating in the gallbladder channel and struggling against vital qi.

Table 9.69 Gallbladder Channel Damp Heat

Common Pathogenesis	
Accumulation of damp heat in the gallbladder	
Manifestations	**Systematic Pathogenesis**
Pain in the right abdomen or right hypochondrium, tenderness	Depression of gallbladder qi
Alternating attacks of fever and chills, or high fever accompanied by shivering due to sensation of cold	Fighting between vital qi and pathogenic factors occurring in the shao yang channel
Yellow greasy tongue coating, bitter taste in mouth, jaundice	Upward steaming of gallbladder heat
Nausea, aggravated by fatty food	Dysfunction of the spleen and stomach
Irregular defecation and dark-colored urine	Downward flow of damp heat
Red tongue and wiry rapid pulse	Damp heat stagnating in the body

Main manifestations: Alternating attacks of fever and chills, or high fever accompanied by shivering due to cold, combined with manifestations as seen in **liver channel damp heat patterns (Table 9.63).**

IX. PATTERN IDENTIFICATION ACCORDING TO THE KIDNEY

The method of pattern identification for disorders of the kidney is based on understanding the physiological functions and pathological characteristics of the kidney. The manifestations obtained from the four diagnostic methods are analyzed in this light and a final pattern diagnosis is achieved.

Kidney disorders mainly involve the functions of the kidney in governing growth and development, reproduction, and metabolism of body fluids, as well as defecation and urination.

1. MAIN ANALYSIS OF DISORDERS OF THE KIDNEY

The common manifestations and pathogenesis for disorders of the kidney are analyzed in Table 9.70.

Table 9.70 Manifestations and Pathogenesis for Disorders of the Kidney

Common Pathogenesis	
Dysfunction in storing kidney essence	
Manifestations	**Systematic Pathogenesis**
Delayed development in physique and intelligence, including the five kinds of retardation in infants (standing, walking, speaking, hair growth, tooth eruption) and the five kinds of flaccidity in infants (flaccidity of the head, neck, extremities, muscles, and mastication); soreness and weakness of lumbar region and knees	Insufficiency of kidney essence leading to poor nourishment and promotion of the body and mind
Sterility or infertility	Deficiency of kidney essence in men; cold accumulating in the uterus in women
Nocturnal emissions	Deficiency of kidney yin leading to the rising of ministerial fire
Premature ejaculation, spermatorrhea, and impotence	Decline of life gate fire brought on by a deficiency of kidney yang
Insomnia, dream-disturbed sleep, deafness, tinnitus, dizziness, vertigo, headache with hollow sensation in head	Poor filling of the reservoir of the marrow leading to poor nourishment of the brain
Common Pathogenesis	
Dysfunction of metabolism of body fluids	
Manifestations	**Systematic Pathogenesis**
Edema	Deficiency of kidney yang leading to dysfunction of the bladder, with body fluids retained in the subcutaneous parts of the body
Retention of urine	Blood stasis or deficiency of kidney yang leading to poor opening and closing of the bladder
Loose stools before dawn, leukorrhea with watery vaginal discharge	Decline of life gate fire leading to poor warmth of the spleen

Diagnosis in Traditional Chinese Medicine

2. COMMON PATTERN TYPES

Most common patterns of kidney disorders are characterized by deficiency.

Kidney Yang Deficiency

This refers to a condition of kidney yang deficiency leading to poor warmth of the body and limbs.

Table 9.71 Kidney Yang Deficiency

Common Pathogenesis	
Insufficiency of kidney yang	
Manifestations	**Systematic Pathogenesis**
Soreness, weakness, and pain of the lumbar region and knees with cold sensation, aversion to cold, cold limbs	Poor warmth of the body and limbs
Pigmented cheeks	Reversal of turbid yin
Impotence, spermatorrhea, premature ejaculation	Decline of life gate fire leading to poor consolidation of semen
Sterility or infertility	Deficient ejaculation for men or poor warming of the uterus for women
Diarrhea before dawn	Decline of life gate fire leading to poor warmth of the spleen
Retention of urine, edema, pale and puffy tongue	Dysfunction of the metabolism of body fluids
Deep and indistinct pulse	Poor promotion of blood circulation

Main manifestations: Hypoactivity of kidney functions and soreness and weakness of the lumbar region, combined with manifestations as seen in **deficiency cold patterns (Table 6.11).**

Kidney Yin Deficiency

This refers to a condition of kidney yin deficiency leading to the production of deficiency fire.

Table 9.72 Kidney Yin Deficiency

Common Pathogenesis	
Insufficiency of kidney yin	
Manifestations	**Systematic Pathogenesis**
Soreness and weakness of the lumbar region and knees	Poor nourishment of the lumbar region
Dizziness, tinnitus, insomnia	Flaring up of deficiency fire
Hyperactivity of sexual function, marked by nocturnal emissions	Stirring up of the ministerial fire
Scant menses, dysmenorrhea	Poor filling of the thoroughfare and controlling channels
Heavy menses	Deficiency fire compressing blood out of the vessels
Malar flush, tidal fever, night sweats, five-palm heat, dry throat and mouth, red tongue with scant coating	Deficiency fire flaring up and consuming body fluids
Thin and rapid pulse	Deficiency fire accumulating in the body

Main manifestations: Soreness and weakness of the lumbar region and knees, hyperactivity of sexual function, and irregular menstruation, combined with manifestations as seen in **yin deficiency patterns (Table 6.10).**

Kidney Essence Deficiency

This refers to a condition of kidney essence deficiency leading to retardation of growth and development or to senility.

Table 9.73 Kidney Essence Deficiency

Common Pathogenesis	
Insufficiency of kidney essence	
Manifestations	**Systematic Pathogenesis**
Soreness and weakness of the lumbar region and knees; poor physical and mental development	Poor nourishment of the skeleton and brain
Senility, premature graying of hair, loss of hair and teeth	Poor nourishment of the hair and teeth

Sterility or infertility	Poor nourishment of the thoroughfare and controlling channels
Pale tongue and deep thin pulse	Poor nourishment and filling of the blood vessels

Main manifestations: Soreness and weakness of the lumbar region and knees, poor physical and mental development, senility, and sterility or infertility.

Kidney Qi Failing to Consolidate

This refers to a condition of kidney qi deficiency leading to a poor consolidation of sperm, menses, urine, stools, and of the fetus (also referred to as "five leaks").

Table 9.74 Kidney Qi Failing to Consolidate

Common Pathogenesis	
Insufficiency of kidney qi	
Manifestations	**Systematic Pathogenesis**
Soreness and weakness of the lumbar region, lassitude, listlessness	Poor promotion of qi and blood circulation to nourish the body
Frequent urination, nocturnal urination, incontinence of urine, bedwetting, enuresis	Poor consolidation of the bladder
Lingering diarrhea, dawn diarrhea, incontinence of stool	Poor consolidation of the large intestine
Spermatorrhea, premature ejaculation	Poor consolidation of semen
Heavy menses, dysfunctional uterine bleeding, watery vaginal discharge	Poor consolidation of the thoroughfare and controlling channels
Habitual miscarriage	Poor consolidation of the fetus
Pale tongue, deep indistinct pulse	Poor promotion and filling of blood circulation

Main manifestations: Soreness and weakness of the lumbar region, and poor consolidation of semen, stools, urine, menses and the fetus, combined with manifestations as seen in **qi deficiency patterns (Table 8.2).**

Kidney Failing to Grasp Qi

This refers to a condition of insufficient kidney qi failing to grasp qi in respiration. The basic clinical manifestations are the same as kidney qi deficiency.

Table 9.75 Kidney Failing to Grasp Qi

Common Pathogenesis	
Decline of kidney qi	
Manifestations	**Systematic Pathogenesis**
Soreness and weakness of the lumbar region and knees	Poor promotion of qi and blood circulation to nourish the body
Asthma with difficulty inhaling, shortness of breath	Inability to grasp the qi brought in by the lung
Weak pulsation at the chi position pulse (both sides)	Poor promotion of blood circulation

Main manifestations: Difficult inhalation, combined with manifestations as seen in **kidney qi failing to consolidate (Table 9.74).**

X. PATTERN IDENTIFICATION ACCORDING TO THE BLADDER

The method of pattern identification for disorders of the bladder is based on understanding the physiological functions and pathological characteristics of the bladder. The manifestations obtained from the four diagnostic methods are analyzed in this light and a final pattern diagnosis is achieved.

Bladder disorders commonly involve the functions of the bladder in storing urine and directing urination. Therefore, they manifest as changes in urination, and, sometimes, as abnormal sensations in the lower abdomen.

The functions of the kidney affect those of the bladder because they are linked in an exterior-interior relationship.

1. MAIN ANALYSIS OF DISORDERS OF THE BLADDER

An analysis of the general manifestations and the pathogenesis for disorders of the bladder is shown in Table 9.76.

Table 9.76 Manifestations and Pathogenesis for Disorders of the Bladder

Common Pathogenesis	
Dysfunction of the bladder in storing urine and directing urination	
Manifestations	**Systematic Pathogenesis**
Frequent urination	Poor consolidation of urine
Enuresis, bedwetting	Poor consolidation of the bladder in opening and closing
Urgent and painful urination	Downward flow of damp heat

Diagnosis in Traditional Chinese Medicine

2. COMMON PATTERN TYPES

Common patterns of bladder disorders include only bladder damp heat and deficiency cold.

Bladder Damp Heat

This refers to a condition of damp heat accumulating in the bladder, leading to the dysfunction of the bladder in closing and opening.

Table 9.77 Bladder Damp Heat

Common Pathogenesis	
Damp heat accumulating in the bladder	
Manifestations	**Systematic Pathogenesis**
Frequent urination	Dysfunction of the bladder
Urgent and painful urination with burning sensation, dark-colored urine	Downward flow of damp heat into the lower burner
Bloody urine	Impairment of blood vessels
Yellow tongue coating, rolling rapid pulse	Damp heat accumulating in the body

Main manifestations: Frequent, urgent, and painful urination with burning sensation, combined with manifestations as seen in **damp patterns (Table 7.4).**

Bladder Deficiency Cold

This refers to a condition of insufficient kidney yang leading to poor warmth of the bladder.

Table 9.78 Bladder Deficiency Cold

Common Pathogenesis	
Insufficiency of kidney yang	
Manifestations	**Systematic Pathogenesis**
Frequent urination with clear urine or bedwetting	Poor warmth leading to lack of consolidation of the bladder
Aversion to cold, cold limbs, lassitude, listlessness	Poor warmth of the whole body
Pale tongue, deep and weak pulse	Poor promotion of blood circulation

Main manifestations: Abnormal urination combined with manifestations as seen in **yang deficiency patterns (Table 6.11).**

XI. IMPORTANT DIFFERENTIAL DIAGNOSES OF PATTERNS ACCORDING TO THE INTERNAL ORGANS

The same type of deficiency can be found in several different disorders of the internal organs, so a differential diagnosis is necessary.

1. YIN DEFICIENCY

Yin deficiency patterns can be found in disorders of the lung, spleen, heart, liver, and kidney.

Table 9.79 Yin Deficiency Patterns

Common Manifestations		Common Pathogenesis	
Tidal fever, malar flush, night sweats, five-palm heat, red tongue with scant coating, thin rapid pulse		Insufficiency of yin fluids leading to production of deficiency heat	
Deficiency Pattern	**Systematic Manifestations**	**Systematic Pathogenesis**	
Lung yin	Dry cough or cough with scant and sticky sputum or coughing blood	Poor nourishment of the lung leading to dysfunction in dispersing and precipitating	
Spleen yin	Poor appetite, abdominal distension, scant saliva, dry mouth and lips	Poor nourishment of the spleen leading to dysfunction in transporting and transforming	
Heart yin	Palpitations, insomnia, dream-disturbed sleep, irritability	Poor nourishment of the heart leading to dysfunction in governing the blood and mind	
Liver yin	Pain in the hypochondrial region with a burning sensation, dryness and discomfort of the eyes	Poor nourishment of the liver leading to dysfunction in spreading and precipitating	
Kidney yin	Hyperactive sexual drive, scant menses, even amenorrhea, or heavy menses, soreness and weakness of the lumbar area and knees	Poor nourishment of the kidney leading to dysfunction in governing reproduction and stirring up ministerial fire	

2. YANG DEFICIENCY

Yang deficiency patterns can be found in disorders of the spleen, heart, and kidney.

Table 9.80 Yang Deficiency

Common Manifestations		Common Pathogenesis
Aversion to cold, cold limbs, lassitude, listlessness, puffy and pale face , tongue with white moist tongue coating, deep slow pulse		Insufficiency of yang leading to poor warmth
Deficiency Pattern	**Differentiating Manifestations**	**Differentiating Pathogenesis**
Spleen yang	Poor appetite, abdominal pain and distension with preference for warmth and pressure, loose stools, edema	Dysfunction in transporting and transforming foodstuff and damp
Heart yang	Palpitations, oppression of the chest, occasional cardiac pain, knotted or intermittent pulse	Dysfunction in promoting blood circulation
Kidney yang	Impotence, premature ejaculation, sterility, frequent urination, enuresis, or retention of urine, diarrhea before dawn, edema	Dysfunction in consolidating the two yin

3. Qi Deficiency

Qi deficiency patterns can be found in disorders of the lung, spleen, heart, and kidney.

Table 9.81 Qi Deficiency

Common Manifestations		Common Pathogenesis
Lassitude, listlessness, shortness of breath, dizziness, spontaneous sweating, pale tongue, and weak pulse, all manifestations worsening after exertion		Insufficiency of qi leading to hypofunction of the internal organs
Deficiency Pattern	**Differentiating Manifestations**	**Differentiating Pathogenesis**
Lung qi	Cough and asthma with weak soft voice, no desire to speak, white thin sputum	Hypofunction in promotion of respiration and voice
Spleen qi	Poor appetite, abdominal distension, loose stools, bruising easily, prolapse of internal organs	Hypofunction in transportation and transformation of foodstuff and damp
Heart qi	Palpitations, oppression of the chest, weak pulse with irregular heartbeat	Hypofunction in promotion of blood circulation and the mind

	Soreness and weakness of lumbar area and knees, long-lasting diarrhea, dawn diarrhea, incontinence of stools; frequent and nocturnal urination, incontinence of urine, bedwetting; seminal emissions; heavy menses and watery vaginal discharge; habitual miscarriage	Hypofunction in consolidation of stools, urine, semen, and of the fetus and menses; vaginal discharge
Kidney qi		

4. BLOOD DEFICIENCY

Blood deficiency patterns can be found in disorders of the heart and liver.

Table 9.82 Blood Deficiency

Common Pathogenesis		Common Manifestations
Insufficiency of blood leading to poor nourishment of the body and limbs		Dim, sallow, or pale complexion, dizziness, pale lips, nails and tongue, numbness of the body and extremities, thin pulse
Deficiency Pattern	Differentiating Pathogenesis	Differentiating Manifestations
Heart blood	Poor nourishment of the heart and mind	Palpitations, insomnia, poor concentration and forgetfulness
Liver blood	Poor nourishment of the tendons, nails, and eyes and poor filling of the thoroughfare and controlling channels	Blurred vision, night blindness, color blindness, floaters; brittle nails, delayed and scant menses light red in color or amenorrhea

XII. COMBINED PATTERNS OF THE INTERNAL ORGANS

Most cases in clinical practice present as combined patterns. These are identified according to the main manifestations of each individual pattern.

1. HEART QI-LUNG QI DEFICIENCY

This pattern is characterized by an insufficiency of heart qi and lung qi, and also manifests as lassitude, listlessness, dizziness, spontaneous sweating, and pale tongue and weak pulse, the common manifestations of **qi deficiency patterns (Table 8.2).**

Table 9.83 Heart Qi-Lung Qi Deficiency Pattern

Common Pathogenesis	
Heart qi deficiency combined with lung qi deficiency	
Manifestations	**Systematic Pathogenesis**
Palpitations, oppression of the chest	Insufficiency of heart qi leading to poor promotion of heart blood
Cough and asthma with weak and soft voice, thin clear sputum	Insufficiency of lung qi leading to poor promotion of respiration and voice

2. LUNG QI-SPLEEN QI DEFICIENCY

This pattern is characterized by an insufficiency of lung qi and spleen qi, and also manifests as lassitude, listlessness, dizziness, spontaneous sweating, pale tongue and weak pulse, the common manifestations of **qi deficiency patterns (Table 8.2).**

Table 9.84 Lung Qi-Spleen Qi Deficiency Pattern

Common Pathogenesis	
Lung qi deficiency combined with spleen qi deficiency	
Manifestations	**Systematic Pathogenesis**
Cough and asthma with weak and soft voice, thin clear sputum	Insufficiency of lung qi leading to poor promotion of respiration and voice
Poor appetite, abdominal distension, loose stools	Insufficiency of spleen qi leading to poor transportation and transformation of food-stuff and damp

3. LUNG QI -KIDNEY QI DEFICIENCY

This pattern is characterized by an insufficiency of lung qi and kidney qi, and also manifests as shortness of breath, lassitude, listlessness, dizziness, spontaneous sweating, and pale tongue and weak pulse, the common manifestations of **qi deficiency patterns (Table 8.2).**

Table 9.85 Lung Qi-Kidney Qi Deficiency Pattern

Common Pathogenesis	
Lung qi deficiency combined with kidney qi deficiency	
Manifestations	**Systematic Pathogenesis**
Cough and asthma with weak and soft voice, thin clear sputum	Insufficiency of lung qi leading to poor promotion of respiration
Asthma with difficult inhalation, soreness and weakness of the lumbar region and knees, chronic diarrhea, dawn diarrhea; bedwetting, frequent and nocturnal urination, seminal emissions; heavy menses, watery leukorrhea; habitual miscarriage	Insufficiency of kidney qi leading to poor consolidation of stools, urine, semen; of the menses and fetus; vaginal discharge

4. HEART BLOOD-LIVER BLOOD DEFICIENCY

This pattern is characterized by an insufficiency of heart blood and liver blood, and also manifests as dizziness, sallow or pale face, lips, tongue and nails, numbness of the body and extremities, and thin pulse, the common manifestations of **blood deficiency patterns (Table 8.6).**

Table 9.86 Heart Blood-Liver Blood Deficiency Pattern

Common Pathogenesis	
Heart blood deficiency combined with liver blood deficiency	
Manifestations	**Systematic Pathogenesis**
Palpitations, insomnia, poor concentration, forgetfulness	Insufficiency of heart blood leading to poor nourishment of the heart and mind
Blurred vision, floaters, night blindness, color blindness, delayed scant menses of a light color or amenorrhea	Insufficiency of liver blood leading to poor nourishment of the eyes and poor filling of the thoroughfare and controlling channels

5. HEART BLOOD-SPLEEN QI DEFICIENCY

This pattern is characterized by an insufficiency of heart blood and spleen qi. Students, academicians, and intellectuals (all those who frequently and actively utilize mental power) tend to have this pattern.

Table 9.87 Heart Blood-Spleen Qi Deficiency

Common Pathogenesis	
Heart blood deficiency combined with spleen qi deficiency	
Manifestations	**Systematic Pathogenesis**
Palpitations, insomnia, poor concentration, forgetfulness	Insufficiency of heart blood leading to poor nourishment of the heart and mind
Poor appetite, abdominal distension, loose stools, bleeding, prolapse of internal organs	Insufficiency of spleen qi leading to poor transportation and transformation of food-stuff and damp

6. LIVER YIN-KIDNEY YIN DEFICIENCY

This pattern is characterized by an insufficiency of liver yin and kidney yin, and also manifests as malar flush, night sweats, five-palm heat, red tongue, and thin rapid pulse, the common manifestations of **yin deficiency patterns (Table 6.10).**

Table 9.88 Liver Yin-Kidney Yin Deficiency Pattern

Common Pathogenesis	
Liver yin deficiency combined with kidney yin deficiency	
Manifestations	**Systematic Pathogenesis**
Discomfort and dry, rough feeling in the eyes, pain of the hypochondrium, irritability	Insufficiency of liver yin leading to poor nourishment of the body and production of deficiency heat
Soreness and weakness of the lumbar region and knees, nocturnal emissions, deafness, tinnitus	Insufficiency of kidney yin leading to poor nourishment of the body and production of deficiency heat

7. LUNG YIN-KIDNEY YIN DEFICIENCY

This pattern is characterized by an insufficiency of lung yin and kidney yin, and also manifests as malar flush, afternoon fevers, night sweats, five-palm heat, red tongue, and thin rapid pulse, the common manifestations of yin deficiency.

Table 9.89 Lung Yin-Kidney Yin Deficiency Pattern

Common Pathogenesis	
Deficiency of lung yin combined with deficiency of kidney yin	
Manifestations	**Systematic Pathogenesis**
Cough with scant sputum and difficult expectoration, possibly coughing blood	Insufficiency of lung yin leading to poor nourishment of the body and production of deficiency heat
Soreness and weakness of the lumbar region and knees, nocturnal emissions, deafness, tinnitus	Insufficiency of kidney yin leading to poor nourishment of the body and production of deficiency heat

8. DISHARMONY BETWEEN THE KIDNEY AND THE HEART

This pattern is characterized by an insufficiency of kidney yin and the upward flaring of heart fire.

Table 9.90 Disharmony between the Kidney and the Heart

Common Pathogenesis	
Kidney yin deficiency combined with heart fire flaring upward	
Manifestations	**Systematic Pathogenesis**
Soreness and weakness of the lumbar region and knees, nocturnal emissions, deafness, tinnitus	Insufficiency of kidney yin leading to weakening of the lower body
Irritability, insomnia, dream-disturbed sleep, sores on tongue body and in the mouth, red tip of the tongue	Loss of control of kidney water leading to upward flaring of heart fire

9. SPLEEN YANG-KIDNEY YANG DEFICIENCY

This pattern is characterized by an insufficiency of spleen yang and kidney yang, and also manifests as aversion to cold, cold limbs, pale puffy tongue with white coating, and deep slow pulse with forceless beat, the common manifestations of **yang deficiency patterns (Table 6.11).**

Table 9.91 Spleen Yang-Kidney Yang Deficiency

Common Pathogenesis	
Spleen yang deficiency combined with kidney yang deficiency	
Manifestations	**Systematic Pathogenesis**
Abdominal pain, preference for warmth and pressure, poor appetite, loose stools, edema	Insufficiency of spleen yang leading to poor transportation and transformation
Pain in the abdomen, lumbar area, and knee with cold sensation, edema with scant urine	Insufficiency of kidney yang leading to poor warmth of the skeleton and poor closing and opening of the bladder

10. HEART YANG-KIDNEY YANG DEFICIENCY

This pattern is characterized by an insufficiency of heart yang and kidney yang, and also manifests as aversion to cold, cold limbs, pale tongue with white coating, and deep slow pulse, the common manifestations of **yang deficiency patterns (Table 6.11).**

Table 9.92 Heart Yang-Kidney Yang Deficiency

Common Pathogenesis	
Heart yang deficiency combined with kidney yang deficiency	
Manifestations	**Systematic Pathogenesis**
Palpitations, occasional sensations of pain and oppression in the cardiac region, somnolence, purple lips and tongue, and choppy pulse	Insufficiency of heart yang leading to poor promotion of the blood circulation
Soreness and weakness of the lumbar region and knees with cold sensation, possibly edema with scant urine	Insufficiency of kidney yang leading to poor warmth of skeleton and poor closing and opening of the bladder

11. LIVER FIRE ATTACKING THE LUNG

This pattern is characterized by the rise of liver fire causing reversal of lung qi.

Table 9.93 Liver Fire Attacking the Lung

Common Pathogenesis	
Liver fire rising and attacking the lung leading to dysfunction of the lung in dispersing and precipitating	
Manifestations	**Systematic Pathogenesis**
Distension and pain of the chest and hypochondrium, irritability, bloodshot eyes	Rising of liver fire leading to qi and blood rushing up
Paroxysmal cough and asthma, aggravated by emotional depression or anger, bloody sputum or coughing blood	Liver fire attacking the lung leading to reversal of lung qi

12. DISHARMONY BETWEEN THE LIVER AND THE SPLEEN

This pattern is characterized by stagnation of liver qi and weakness of spleen qi.

Table 9.94 Disharmony between the Liver and the Spleen

Common Pathogenesis	
Liver qi stagnation combined with spleen qi deficiency	
Manifestations	**Systematic Pathogenesis**
Emotional depression, frequent sighing, irritability, distension and fullness of the hypochondrium, and wiry pulse	Liver qi stagnation leading to poor spreading and precipitating
Poor appetite, abdominal pain, loose stools, or irritable bowel movements, defecation with discomfort of the anus	Liver qi overstimulating the spleen leading to poor transportation and transformation of foodstuff and damp

13. DISHARMONY BETWEEN THE LIVER AND THE STOMACH

This pattern is characterized by stagnation of liver qi and reversal of stomach qi.

Table 9.95 Disharmony between the Liver and the Stomach

Common Pathogenesis	
Liver qi stagnation combined with stomach qi reversal	
Manifestations	**Systematic Pathogenesis**
Emotional depression, frequent sighing, irritability, distension and fullness of the hypochondrium, wiry pulse	Liver qi stagnation leading to poor dispersing and precipitating functions of the liver
Nausea, vomiting, belching, hiccups, acid reflux; aggravated by emotional distress	Liver qi transversely attacking the stomach leading to reversal of stomach qi

14. LIVER AND GALLBLADDER DAMP HEAT

This pattern is characterized by damp heat from both the liver and gallbladder, and manifests as yang-type jaundice.

Table 9.96 Liver and Gallbladder Damp Heat

Common Pathogenesis	
Damp heat accumulating in the liver and gallbladder leading to dysfunction of the liver and gallbladder in dispersing and descending	
Manifestations	**Systematic Pathogenesis**
Distending pain of the hypochondrium, tension, abdominal distension, wiry rapid pulse	Damp heat disturbing the flow of liver qi
Poor appetite, nausea, vomiting, yellow greasy tongue coating	Damp heat disturbing the flow of stomach qi
Jaundice with bright yellow coloration of the skin, eyes, and urine	Damp heat disturbing the drainage of bile

15. SPLEEN AND STOMACH COLD DAMP

This pattern has the characteristics of cold damp from the spleen and stomach, and manifests as yin-type jaundice.

Table 9.97 Spleen and Stomach Cold Damp

Common Pathogenesis	
Cold damp accumulating in the middle burner leading to poor digestion	
Manifestations	**Systematic Pathogenesis**
Distension and fullness of the upper abdomen, poor appetite, white greasy tongue coating, soft slow pulse	Cold damp accumulating in the spleen and inhibiting the spleen's functions of transportation and transformation
Nausea, vomiting of thin clear saliva	Cold damp accumulating in the stomach leading to reversal of stomach qi
Loose stools, heaviness of the head and whole body	Downward flow of cold damp
Jaundice with dim yellow-colored skin and eyes	Cold damp disturbing the drainage of bile

CHAPTER TEN

Pattern Identification According to the Six Channels

This method of pattern identification analyzes the manifestations of a disease and confirms the diagnosis by using the tai yang, shao yang, yang ming, tai yin, shao yin, and jue yin channels as the guiding principles, with each channel representing a different stage in the development of the disease. Pattern identification according to the six channels is commonly used to identify disorders caused by the six environmental pathogenic factors.

I. MAIN PATTERN TYPES

The main patterns are named after the six channels, and are divided into three yang patterns (tai yang, shao yang, and yang ming) and three yin patterns (tai yin, shao yin, and jue yin). The yang channel patterns concern tai yang, shao yang, and yang ming patterns, while the three yin channel patterns relate to tai yin, shao yin, and jue yin patterns.

1. TAI YANG PATTERNS

Tai yang patterns are classified into two basic categories, tai yang channel patterns and tai yang bowel patterns. Of the three yang channels the tai yang channel is the first to be attacked by external pathogens.

Tai Yang Channel Patterns

A tai yang channel pattern is caused by pathogenic wind cold attacking the exterior of the body. When the ying and wei systems are struggling to defend the body against attacks of wind cold, the resultant condition is a tai yang pattern. Tai yang channel patterns manifest as exterior cold patterns and indicate the early stage of febrile diseases.

Table 10.1 Tai Yang Channel Patterns due to Wind

Common Pathogenesis	
Wind attacking the exterior of the body	
Manifestations	**Systematic Pathogenesis**
Fever, floating pulse	Fighting between vital qi and pathogens occurring in the exterior of the body
Aversion to wind, moderate floating pulse	Loose muscular interstices
Sweating	Poor consolidation leading to disharmony between ying and wei levels

Table 10.2 Tai Yang Channel Patterns due to Cold

Common Pathogenesis	
Cold attacking the exterior of the body	
Manifestations	**Systematic Pathogenesis**
Chills, absence of sweat	The wei qi is being restrained in the interior of the body by pathogenic cold, leading to insufficient warming of the body surface
Fever	Fighting between vital qi and pathogens occurring in the exterior of the body
Floating tense pulse	Cold contracts the blood vessels, leading to a tense pulse, while a floating pulse indicates an exterior condition.

Tai Yang Bowel Patterns

A tai yang bowel pattern occurs when a tai yang channel pattern is not relieved and the pathogens subsequently penetrate the tai yang bowel (bladder) channel. This condition may be characterized by water retention or blood stagnation.

Table 10.3 Tai Yang Bowel Patterns due to Water Retention

Common Pathogenesis	
Invading pathogens lead to water accumulating in the bladder	
Manifestations	**Systematic Pathogenesis**
Chills, fever, floating or rapid floating pulse	External pathogens remaining in the exterior of the body
Oliguria, lower abdominal distension	Dysfunction of the opening and closing of the bladder orifice leading to water remaining in the lower burner
Thirst with vomiting after drinking fluids	Water retention due to inability of body fluids to steam upwards

Table 10.4 Tai Yang Bowel Patterns due to Blood Stagnation

Common Pathogenesis	
Pathogenic heat accumulating in the lower abdomen with blood stasis	
Manifestations	**Systematic Pathogenesis**
Severe pain in the lower abdomen	Restraint of wei qi leading to an obstruction of qi and blood circulation
Mental confusion, including mania and forgetfulness	Accumulated heat disturbing the mind
Normal urination	Disorder occurring in the blood system that does not involve bladder qi
Tar-like stools	Stagnated blood excreted with stools
Deep choppy or knotted pulse	Accumulated heat leading to a blockage of blood circulation

2. YANG MING PATTERNS

Yang ming patterns are caused by excess heat from the stomach and large intestine, and indicate a fully manifested febrile disease.

Yang ming patterns are divided into two categories: yang ming channel patterns and the yang ming bowel patterns. At this stage, both categories indicate heat that is penetrating into the interior. This is usually derived from a tai yang pattern that has worsened due to a lack of or inappropriate medical treatment. The distinguishing factor between yang ming channel and bowel patterns is that in yang ming channel patterns, excess heat is steaming and spreading over the entire body, whereas in yang ming bowel patterns, excess heat is combined with dry stools accumulating in the yang ming bowel and manifests as severe constipation.

Yang Ming Channel Patterns

A yang ming channel pattern is caused by excess heat that remains in the yang ming channel and spreads over the entire body.

Table 10.5 Yang Ming Channel Pattern

Common Pathogenesis	
Excess heat accumulating in the interior of the body	
Manifestations	**Systematic Pathogenesis**
High fever, dry yellow tongue coating	Internal heat dispersing outward
Profuse sweating	Body fluids pressing outwards
Severe thirst with urgent desire to intake fluids	Impairment of body fluids
Irritability	Upward flaring of excess heat affecting the mind
Flooding pulse	Promotion of blood circulation

Yang Ming Bowel Patterns

Yang ming bowel patterns refer to conditions in which excess heat combined with dry stool accumulates in the large intestine, resulting in severe constipation.

Table 10.6 Yang Ming Bowel Patterns

Common Pathogenesis	
Deep-seated heat in the yang ming bowel	
Manifestations	**Systematic Pathogenesis**
Tidal fever aggravated in the afternoon	Heat dispersing outward when yang ming qi is rising
Constipation, fullness, tenderness, and distending pain of the abdomen	Accumulation of both excess heat and dry stools leading to an obstruction of stomach and large intestine qi
Red tongue with yellow dry coating	Impairment of body fluids
Deep or deep slow pulse with forceful beats	Excess heat constrained in the interior of the body

Diagnosis in Traditional Chinese Medicine

3. SHAO YANG PATTERNS

A shao yang pattern is caused by pathogens attacking the shao yang bowel (gallbladder) and disrupting the gallbladder's dispersing function. This pattern is located between the exterior and interior of the body, and is known as the half exterior-half interior pattern. Shao yang patterns are most notably marked by alternating attacks of chills and fever and may also result from the transmission of a tai yang pattern to the interior. In this pattern, fevers result when the vital qi is strong and is successfully fighting pathogens; chills result when the pathogens increase in strength and dominate the opposing qi.

Table 10.7 Shao Yang Patterns

Common Pathogenesis	
External pathogens invading the area of the body that is half exterior and half interior	
Manifestations	**Systematic Pathogenesis**
Alternating attacks of chills and fever	Pathogens fighting with vital qi in the area between the interior and exterior
Fullness and distension of the hypochondrium and abdomen	Stagnation of qi along the jue yin channel which is in an interior-exterior relation with shao yang
Poor appetite, nausea, vomiting, wiry pulse	Stagnation of gallbladder qi leading to stomach qi reversal
Irritability	Excess heat accumulating in the interior of the body
Bitter taste in mouth, dry throat, dizziness	Gallbladder qi steaming upward

4. TAI YIN PATTERNS

A tai yin pattern is caused by insufficient spleen qi producing cold damp, thus creating an interior deficiency cold pattern. This pattern may be caused by injured spleen qi due to inappropriate medical treatment in the three yang channels or by pathogenic cold directly attacking a tai yin channel. A tai yin pattern is characterized by a preexisting spleen qi deficiency which further impairs the transformation and transportation process, and leads to the retention of cold damp. When pathogenic factors invade the three yin channels, the tai yin channel is the first to be attacked.

Table 10.8 Tai Yin Patterns

Common Pathogenesis	
External pathogenic invastion combined with spleen deficiency leading to the production of cold damp	
Manifestations	**Systematic Pathogenesis**
Fullness of the abdomen, vomiting, poor appetite	Poor transportation and transformation function of the spleen
Loose stools	Dysfunction in lifting lucid yang
Abdominal pain relieved by warmth and pressure	Poor warmth of the abdomen
No desire to drink fluids, pale tongue with white coating, slow pulse	Cold damp accumulating in the body

5. SHAO YIN PATTERNS

Shao yin patterns are caused by a chronic illness or inappropriate medical treatment that has injured kidney and heart yang or kidney and heart yin. Shao yin patterns occur during the late stage of a febrile disease. They are classified as either shao yin cold patterns or shao yin heat patterns, presenting as insufficiency of yang for the cold type and insufficiency of yin for the heat type.

Shao Yin Cold Patterns

Shao yin cold patterns are characterized by an insufficiency of heart and kidney yang.

Table 10.9 Shao Yin Cold Pattern

Common Pathogenesis	
Insufficiency of heart yang combined with insufficiency of kidney yang leading to poor warmth of the body	
Manifestations	**Systematic Pathogenesis**
Somnolence	Poor invigoration of the mind
Aversion to cold, cold limbs, lassitude, listlessness	Poor warmth of the entire body
Chronic loose stools or dawn diarrhea	Poor promotion of intestinal qi
No desire to drink fluids	No impairment of body fluids
Pale tongue and deep slow pulse	Poor promotion of blood circulation

Shao Yin Heat Patterns

Shao yin heat patterns are characterized by an insufficiency of heart and kidney yin.

Table 10.10 Shao Yin Heat Pattern

Common Pathogenesis	
Heart yin deficiency combined with kidney yin deficiency leading to poor nourishment of the body and deficiency heat	
Manifestations	**Systematic Pathogenesis**
Insomnia, irritability, five-palm heat	Heart fire flaring up and stirring the mind
Night sweats	Deficiency heat steaming body fluids outward
Dry mouth and throat	Impairment of body fluids
Red tongue tip or dark red or purple tongue with scant coating, thin rapid pulse	Deficiency heat accumulating in the body

6. JUE YIN PATTERNS

Traditionally, jue yin patterns refer to febrile diseases in their most complex and final stage. They are usually transferred from other channel patterns, particularly from lesser yang patterns. Jue yin patterns are marked by heat accumulating in the upper body involving the pericardium and liver, and cold accumulating in the lower body involving the spleen and kidney.

Table 10.11 Jue Yin Pattern

Common Pathogenesis	
Dysfunction of the liver in dispersing and spreading	
Manifestations	**Systematic Pathogenesis**
Fullness in the upper abdomen or a sensation of gas rumbling upward (running piglet qi)	Stagnated liver qi attacking the stomach leading to reversal of stomach qi
Pain in the upper abdomen with a burning sensation, thirst with an urgent desire for fluids	Upward flaring of heat from the pericardium and liver that consumes body fluids
No desire for food; if forced to eat, the patient may regurgitate the food and possibly round worms as well	Liver-spleen disharmony leading to poor regulation of stomach qi
Diarrhea	Cold from the kidney leading to poor warmth of the spleen
Cold limbs	Separation of yin fluids and yang qi

II. RULES FOR TRANSMISSIONS OF THE SIX CHANNEL PATTERNS

Six channel disorders reflect pathogenic changes between the internal organs and the channels. Owing to the relationship between the internal organs and the channels, six channel disorders can transmit from one to another. Rules for transmissions among six channel patterns are as follows:

1. CHUAN JING (TRANSMISSION ALONG THE CHANNELS)

Chuan jing refers to the rules by which pathogens give rise to different patterns by transmitting along different channels. In the beginning, pathogens attack the exterior along a particular channel for which the pattern is named. As the invading pathogens gradually reach the interior of the body, the pathogens transfer to a different channel leading to another pattern which is named for this different channel.

Chuan jing is divided into favorable transmission and unfavorable transmission. Favorable transmission means that the invading pathogens are transmitted along the six channels in the sequence of tai yang→yang ming→shao yang→tai yin→shao yin→jue yin. An unfavorable transmission refers to a progression where pathogens skip from one channel to another, for instance tai yang→tai yin, or yang ming→shao yin. In clinical practice, the patient's constitution or inappropriate medical treatment are commonly seen reasons for an unfavorable transmission. For instance, the inappropriate use of *Da Cheng Qi Tang (Major Qi-Coordinating Decoction)* may cause the transmission of a yang ming bowel pattern into a shao yin cold pattern after severe diarrhea.

2. HE BING (SIMULTANEOUS TRANSMISSION ALONG TWO OR THREE CHANNELS)

He bing refers to the pathogenic condition in which disorders present in a simultaneous two or three channel combination. It means that two or three different channel patterns manifest at the same time.

For instance, at the beginning of an exogenous pathogen-based disease, the patient may manifest tai yang channel pattern and shao yang channel pattern in combination, or shao yang channel pattern and yang ming bowel pattern in combination.

3. BIN BING (INITIAL SEQUENTIAL TRANSMISSION LEADING TO SIMULTANEOUS TRANSMISSION)

Bin bing refers to the pathogenic condition in which one channel pattern initially is secondary to another one which has not improved, until, finally, both channel patterns manifest at the same time.

For instance, a tai yang channel pattern may cause a yang channel pattern. If a tai yang channel pattern still exists when a yang ming channel pattern starts, the patient may manifest exterior cold signs and the "four greatnesses"— great heat, great sweating, great thirst, and great pulse—at the same time.

4. ZHI ZHONG (TRANSMISSION DIRECTLY TO A YIN CHANNEL)

Zhi zhong refers to a pathogenic condition in which one or two, or all three yin channels are attacked directly by the pathogenic factors without transmission via the three yang channels. The patient presents yin channel patterns from the beginning of the disorder.

This is determined by the patient's constitution. For instance, a patient may manifest cold damp in the spleen, indicating a tai yin pattern, without showing any yang channel symptoms, at the beginning of an illness.

CHAPTER ELEVEN

Pattern Identification According to Wei, Qi, Ying, and Blood

This method of pattern identification analyzes the manifestations of a disease and confirms the diagnosis of a pattern by using wei, qi, ying, and blood as the guiding principles. This method is commonly used for pattern identification in warm diseases (epidemic diseases).

The four patterns in this method represent the four stages of a warm disease, namely wei level pattern, qi level pattern, ying (nutrient) level pattern, and blood level pattern. In TCM tradition, warm diseases progress sequentially through wei→qi→ying→blood levels, although, in clinical practice they do not necessarily begin with or follow the perfect order of wei→qi→ying→blood.

I. MAIN PATTERN TYPES

1. WEI LEVEL PATTERN

Wei level patterns are caused by pathogens attacking the lung and the exterior of the body, causing a dysfunction of lung qi and wei qi.

Wei level pattern indicates the early stage of a warm disease and is marked by headache and sore throat. It is combined with manifestations as seen in exterior heat patterns.

Table 11.1 Wei Level Pattern

Common Pathogenesis	
Warm heat attacking the exterior of the body	
Manifestations	**Systematic Pathogenesis**
Fever, slight chills, and thin yellow tongue coating	Stagnation of wei qi occurring on the surface of the body
Headache, sore throat	Upward stirring of heat
Cough	Dysfunction of the lung in dispersing and precipitating qi
Rapid floating pulse	Vital qi struggling against external pathogens on the exterior of the body

2. QI LEVEL PATTERN

Qi level pattern indicates a fully manifested warm disease, and is marked by pathogenic excess heat accumulating in the interior of the body. A qi level pattern presents with a high fever, profuse sweating, severe thirst and a flooding pulse, combined with manifestations of excess heat pattern.

Table 11.2 Qi Level Pattern

Common Pathogenesis	
Excess heat accumulating in the interior of the body	
Manifestations	**Systematic Pathogenesis**
High fever, red tongue with yellow coating	Extreme heat steaming outward
Profuse sweating	Internal heat pressing body fluids outward
Severe thirst with urgent desire for cold drinks, scant and dark colored urine	Heat impairing body fluids
Flooding, rolling, and rapid pulse	Internal heat promoting blood circulation

3. YING LEVEL PATTERN

Ying level pattern is a condition in which pathogens penetrate the pericardium and stir upwards, impairing yin fluids and affecting the mind. Therefore, it manifests as mental disturbance such as insomnia, delirium, loss of consciousness, and a dark red tongue, combined with manifestations seen in excess heat pattern.

Table 11.3 Ying Level Pattern

Common Pathogenesis	
Heat penetrating the pericardium	
Manifestations	**Systematic Pathogenesis**
Fever aggravated at night, not relieved until morning	Impairment of ying yin
Irritability, insomnia, delirium, and possibly loss of consciousness	Pathogens penetrating the pericardium and stirring upwards affecting the mind
Dark red or purple tongue, thin rapid pulse	Extreme heat accompanied by yin deficiency in the ying level

4. BLOOD LEVEL PATTERN

A blood level pattern is a condition in which pathogens profoundly affect the yin and blood systems, involving the heart, the liver, and the kidney. This condition therefore leads to mental disturbance, liver wind, and various kinds of bleeding.

Blood level pattern is the last level of warm disease and, in clinical practice, is often seen in conjunction with a ying level pattern.

Table 11.4 Blood Level Pattern

Common Pathogenesis	
Heat entering the blood level	

Manifestations	Systematic Pathogenesis
Fever aggravated at night, not relieved until morning	Impairment of yin fluids
Severe irritability, delirium, and possibly loss of consciousness	Heat stirring the mind
Petechia or ecchymosis, hematemesis, epistaxis, hematochezia	Extreme heat excessively promoting blood circulation, causing extravasation
Convulsions, opisthotonos, or tremors of the limbs	Extreme heat inducing an attack of liver wind
Dark red or purple tongue, thin rapid pulse	Extreme heat impairing yin fluids with deficiency in the blood level

5. POINTS FOR ATTENTION

Wei, qi, ying, and blood refer to four physical layers in the human body, moving from the exterior to the interior.

Wei, qi, ying, and blood level patterns refer to the four stages of warm disease, progressing from the early stage to the late stage. Clinically, the pathogens may not follow the prescribed sequence of wei, qi, ying, and blood.

The characteristics of four level patterns are seen in Table 11.5 below.

Table 11.5 Characteristics of Four Level Patterns of Warm Disease

Pattern	Location	Characteristics	Manifestations	Stage of Warm Disease
Wei level	Lung and exterior	Exterior heat signs	Chills and fever, head-ache, sore throat, red tongue tip with yellow thin tongue coating, floating rapid pulse	Early
Qi level	Chest, diaphragm, stomach, intestines, gallbladder	Interior heat signs	High fever, profuse sweating, severe thirst, flooding rapid pulse	Middle
Ying level	Pericardium	Mental confusion	Fever aggravated at night, irritability, even delirium, loss of con-sciousness, dark red tongue without coating, thin and rapid pulse	Late
Blood level	Heart, liver, kidney	Wind signs and bleeding	Fever aggravated at night, irritability, bleed-ing, weak hearing, five-palm fever, convulsions or tremors of the fingers and toes	Late

At the blood level, a patient may be affected by two types of liver wind, namely excess liver wind and deficiency liver wind. The excess wind type is caused by extreme heat, whereas deficiency wind is mainly caused by liver yin deficiency. Liver wind due to extreme heat comes from pathogenic heat traveling through the wei, qi, and ying levels. Deficiency wind is caused by the consumption of body fluids leading to liver yin deficiency. Different patients with the same disorder may manifest either one of these types of liver wind depending on the patient's condition. If pathogenic heat is very strong when it reaches the blood level, it will lead to liver wind of the excess type. If the pathogenic heat is not very strong but the body fluid consump-tion is very severe, the result will be liver wind of the deficiency type.

A comparison of liver wind due to extreme heat and liver yin deficiency, as seen in the late stage of a warm disease, is displayed in Table 11.6.

Table 11.6 Comparison of Liver Wind from Extreme Heat and Liver Yin Deficiency

Patterns	Liver Wind Due to Extreme heat	Liver Wind Due to Liver Yin Deficiency
Fever	High fever	Afternoon fever aggravated at night
Mental condition	Mental confusion	Listlessness
Wind signs	Stiff neck, body convulsions, limb spasms, clenched teeth and fists	Trembling of fingers and toes

II. TRANSMISSIONS AMONG THE FOUR LEVEL PATTERNS

Regular transmissions of the four levels are shown below. Complex transmissions among the four levels are shown in Table 11.8.

Table 11.7 Regular Transmissions of the Four Levels

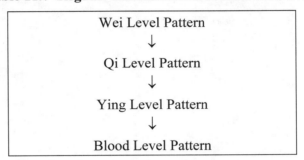

Wei Level Pattern
↓
Qi Level Pattern
↓
Ying Level Pattern
↓
Blood Level Pattern

Table 11.8 Complex Transmissions among the Four Levels

Combined Wei-Qi Level Patterns	At the onset of a warm disease, a patient may be affected by a combined level pattern. Qi level pattern signs may appear at an early stage of a warm disease along with the wei level pattern.
Combined Wei-Ying Level Patterns	This refers to the condition in which epidemic pathogens penetrate the pericardium and cause mental confusion before the wei level pattern is relieved.
Combined Qi-Ying Level Patterns	This refers to the condition in which a qi level pattern marked by the four greatnesses and a ying level pattern marked by mental confusion exist at the same time.
Combined Qi-Blood Level Patterns	This refers to the condition in which wind signs and bleeding start before the four greatnesses are relieved.

CHAPTER TWELVE

Pattern Identification According to Upper, Middle, and Lower Burner

This type of pattern identification analyzes disease manifestations and confirms pattern diagnosis by using the upper burner, middle burner, and lower burner as the guiding principles. This method is commonly used for pattern identification in warm diseases.

The main patterns include upper burner pattern, middle burner pattern, and lower burner pattern, which represent the three stages of a warm disease.

I. MAIN PATTERN TYPES

1. UPPER BURNER PATTERN

Upper burner patterns affect the lung and pericardium and are caused by pathogens attacking these organs. An upper burner pattern refers to the early stage of a warm disease. Mild cases are marked by manifestations as seen in exterior heat patterns and wind heat attacking the lung patterns, while severe cases manifest as heat penetrating the pericardium.

Table 12.1 Upper Burner Pattern (Mild Cases)

Common Pathogenesis	
Warm heat attacking the lung	
Manifestations	**Systematic Pathogenesis**
Fever, slight chills, cough, red tip of the tongue with thin yellow coating, floating and rapid pulse or flooding at the *cun* (inch) position on both sides	Pathogens staying in the exterior of the body leading to dysfunction of the lung in dispersing and precipitating
Headache, sore throat	Warm heat stirring up
Thirst	Warm heat consuming body fluids
Cough and asthma	Reversal of lung qi

Table 12.2 Upper Burner Pattern (Severe Cases)

Common Pathogenesis	
Warm heat penetrating the pericardium	
Manifestations	**Systematic Pathogenesis**
High fever	Pathogenic heat steaming outward
Irritability, delirium, loss of consciousness, stiff tongue with difficulty speaking	Upward stirring of pathogenic heat affecting the mind
Cold limbs	Pathogenic heat restricting yang qi inside, leading to an inability to warm the limbs
Dark red tongue	Pathogenic heat impairing yin fluids

2. MIDDLE BURNER PATTERN

A middle burner pattern indicates the middle stage of a warm disease when pathogenic warm heat affects the middle burner. Based upon the patient's constitution, pathogenic warm heat may transform into yang type dryness with manifestations of pathogenic heat consuming the yin fluids of the stomach and large intestine, or it may transform into yin-type damp with manifestations as seen in damp heat of the spleen.

Middle burner patterns are located in the stomach, large intestine, and spleen.

Table 12.3 Middle Burner Pattern (Yang Type)

Common Pathogenesis	
Warm heat accumulating in the stomach and large intestine transforming into yang-type dryness	
Manifestations	**Systematic Pathogenesis**
High fever, flushed face, deep pulse with forceful beating	Pathogenic heat steaming outward and upward
Fullness and abdominal distension with constipation	Pathogenic heat impairing the body fluids, leading to poor moisture of the intestinal tract
Severe thirst with an urgent desire for cold drinks, dry cracked lips, scant dark urine, red tongue with yellow dry coating or of dark brown color with papillae	Pathogenic heat impairing the body fluids
Irritability, delirium, even loss of consciousness	Upward stirring of pathogenic heat affecting the mind

Diagnosis in Traditional Chinese Medicine

Table 12.4 Middle Burner Pattern (Yin Type)

Common Pathogenesis	
Warm heat accumulating in the spleen transforming into yin-type dampness	
Manifestations	**Systematic Pathogenesis**
Tidal low-grade fever	Pathogenic heat restricted by damp and unable to steam outward
Fullness and distension of the chest and upper abdomen	Damp heat accumulating in the middle burner leading to spleen and stomach qi stagnation
Heaviness of the head and body	Damp heat obstructing channel and collateral qi
Red tongue with yellow greasy coating, soggy and rapid pulse	Damp heat accumulating in the interior of the body

3. LOWER BURNER PATTERN

Lower burner pattern indicates the late stage of a warm disease, and is a condition in which pathogenic heat affects the lower burner and impairs liver and kidney yin. Lower burner patterns affect the liver and kidney.

Table 12.5 Lower Burner Pattern

Common Pathogenesis	
Warm heat entering the lower burner and impairing liver and kidney yin	
Manifestations	**Systematic Pathogenesis**
Tidal fever, malar flush, five-palm heat, dry mouth and throat	Deficiency heat consuming body fluids
Weak hearing	Kidney yin deficiency leading to poor nourishment of the ears
Lassitude, listlessness, possible fainting, dark red tongue with scant coating, weak pulse,	Exhaustion of yin fluids
Twitching or tremors of the limbs	Liver yin deficiency leading to liver wind
Floating and rapid pulse with forceless beating	Poor filling of the blood vessels and poor promotion of blood circulation

4. CHARACTERISTICS OF THREE BURNER PATTERNS

The characteristics of three burner patterns, including their location, pathogenesis, and stages, are shown in Table 12.6.

Table 12.6 Characteristics of Three Burner Patterns

Pattern	Location	Pathogenesis	Stage of Warm Disease
Upper Burner	Lung (with favorable transmission)	Warm pathogens attacking the lung	Early stage (mild case)
	Pericardium (with un-favorable transmission)	Warm pathogens penetrating the pericardium	Early stage (severe case)
Middle Burner	Stomach (with constitutional heat in yang ming)	Warm pathogens entering yang ming leading to yang-type dryness	Middle stage interior heat condition
	Spleen (with constitutional damp in tai yin)	Warm pathogens entering tai yin leading to yin-type damp	Damp warm condition
Lower Burner	Liver	Warm pathogens consuming liver and kidney yin	Late stage
	Kidney		

Table 12.7 Rules for Transmissions of Three Burner Patterns

Transmission Type	Pattern	Pathogenesis
Favorable Transmission	Upper burner (lung, exterior of the body)→middle burner (stomach, large intestine, spleen)→lower burner (liver, kidney)	Warm pathogens attacking the body from the exterior to the interior, and from the upper down to the lower
Unfavorable Transmission	From the lung and exterior of the body to the pericardium	Mental confusion with high fever follows exterior heat
Other Transmission Types	Upper burner-middle burner pattern in combination.	Exterior heat coexisting simultaneously with interior heat or damp heat
	Upper burner-lower burner pattern in combination	Exterior heat coexisting simultaneously with kidney yin deficiency
	Middle burner-lower burner pattern in combination	Interior heat in the stomach and large intestine combined with liver and kidney yin deficiency
	Lower burner pattern at the beginning of a warm disease	Liver yin and kidney yin deficiency are present at the beginning of a warm disease.
	Upper burner, middle burner, and lower burner patterns in combination	Warm pathogens spread over the three burners.

CHAPTER THIRTEEN

Discussion of Case Studies

The fourteen case studies discussed here allow the reader to review pattern diagnosis by applying the different methods of pattern identification introduced above.

1. Qi Fall

Patient and Complaint: A 12-year-old male presents at the clinic with complaints of recurring diarrhea over a period of two years and recurring prolapse of the rectum over the past two months.

Interrogation: He reports having loose stools, a condition which had previously been diagnosed as "poor digestion" and for which the prescribed treatment had been ineffective. He states that the symptoms have become more severe. The prolapse of the rectum initially occurred two months ago and has become recurrent with accompanying lassitude and dizziness. He also reports poor appetite, abdominal distension, and a downbearing sensation in the abdomen.

Inspection: Pale face, pale tongue with white coating.

Palpation and Pulse Examination: Thin pulse with forceless beat.

Auscultation and Olfaction: No indications detected.

Pattern Identification: Spleen qi fall pattern.

Explanation: Chronic loose stools have impaired spleen qi, leading to failure to raise lucid yang. Lassitude, dizziness, pale face and tongue, and weak pulse are caused by qi deficiency leading to poor promotion and nourishment of the body. Prolapse of the rectum is brought about by the fall of central qi leading to poor consolidation of the internal organs.

Diagnostic Disease Name: Diarrhea, prolapse of the rectum.

2. Qi Stagnation

Patient and Complaint: A 55-year-old male presents at the clinic with complaints of recurring distension under the right hypochondrium over a period of two years.

Interrogation: He reports having been troubled by distension of the right hypochondrium which radiates to the upper abdomen and is relieved by lying down. Additionally, he reports frequent bouts of sighing and anger, and sticky stools with discomfort of the anus after defecation. This was previously diagnosed as "chronic persistent hepatitis."

Inspection: Red tongue with thin greasy coating.

Palpation and Pulse Examination: Pain in the upper abdomen when pressing and tapping. Slight wiry pulse with forceful beating.

Auscultation and Olfaction: No indications detected.

Pattern Identification: Liver qi stagnation pattern.

Explanation: Recurring distension under the right hypochondrium radiating to the upper abdomen is caused by qi stagnation leading to poor digestion. Frequent sighing and anger are due to liver failing in its function of dispersing and precipitating. Tenderness is due to qi stagnation followed by blood stasis. Sticky stools with discomfort of the anus after defecation is brought about by stagnation of liver qi leading to liver-spleen disharmony and production of dampness. Red tongue with thin greasy coating and wiry pulse support the diagnosis of qi stagnation pattern.

Diagnostic Disease Name: Hypochondrium pain.

3. Wind-Water Attacking the Lung

Patient and Complaint: A 22-year-old male presents at the clinic having suffered from general edema for half a month.

Interrogation: He reports having had a common cold two weeks ago, followed by sudden edema that started with the eyelids and then spread through the whole body, with accompanying high blood pressure. Laboratory urinalysis shows proteinuria and hematuria. This was previously diagnosed as "acute nephritis." He also reports headaches, oliguria, scant urine, and cough.

Inspection: Upon examination, the patient was found to have severe edema of the face and limbs and a thin white tongue coating.

Palpation and Pulse Examination: Pitting edema around both ankles, floating wiry pulse.

Auscultation and Olfaction: No indications detected.

Pattern Identification: Wind-water attacking the lung.

Explanation: The suddenness of the attack, plus the fact that the edema started with the eyelids and was secondary to a common cold, show that the disorder is occurring in the exterior. Severe general edema is brought about by wind attacking the exterior of the body. Scant urine is caused by wind attacking the lung leading to an obstruction of the water passages. Headache, cough, thin tongue coating and floating pulse indicate wind attacking the exterior of the body.

Diagnostic Disease Name: Edema.

4. Upward Flaring of Stomach Fire

Patient and Complaint: A 45-year-old female presents at the clinic complaining of toothache lasting for one month.

Interrogation: She reports that she has suffered from this condition for one month and that both analgesic and anti-inflammatory treatments have been ineffective.

Inspection: Redness and swelling of the gums, thin yellow tongue coating.

Auscultation and Olfaction: Bad breath.

Palpation and Pulse Examination: Wiry rolling pulse.

Pattern Identification: Excess stomach heat.

Explanation: Chronic toothache is due to excess stomach fire accumulating in the interior leading to stagnation of qi and blood. Redness and swelling of the gums is caused by excess stomach fire accumulating in the interior and flaring up. Bad breath is due to adverse upward steaming of turbid stomach qi. Thin yellow tongue coating and wiry rolling pulse are caused by excess heat accumulating in the interior of the body.

Diagnostic Disease Name: Toothache.

5. Heart Qi-Lung Qi Deficiency

Patient and Complaint: A 65-year-old male presents at the clinic with complaints of palpitations, oppression of the chest, asthma, and cough.

Interrogation: He reports that his symptoms of recurring cough, sputum, shortness of breath, and oppression of the chest, which have affected him for more than 20 years, have been variously diagnosed as "chronic bronchitis," "pulmonary emphysema," and "pulmonary heart disease." In recent years, the palpitations, shortness of breath, and oppression of the chest have felt more severe, and have been aggravated by exercise and accompanied by spontaneous sweating and dizziness.

Inspection: Pale face with puffy eyelids, white thin sputum, pale tongue with ecchymosis and petechia along the edge, white greasy tongue coating.

Pulse Feeling: Deep thin and knotted pulse.

Auscultation and Olfaction: Cough with low voice, wheezing sound in the throat.

Pattern Identification: Heart qi-lung qi deficiency pattern.

Explanation: Chronic illness is consuming lung qi. Recurrent cough, shortness of breath and oppression of the chest, aggravated by exercise, is caused by lung qi deficiency leading to poor promotion of sound production. Spontaneous sweating is due to qi deficiency leading to poor consolidation of muscular interstices. Palpitations and dizziness are due to heart qi deficiency leading to poor tonification of the mind. Pale face and tongue are due to qi deficiency leading to poor promotion of blood circulation. Ecchymosis and petechia along the edge of the tongue are due to heart qi deficiency leading to blood stasis.

Diagnostic Disease Name: Palpitations.

6. Lung Qi-Spleen Qi Deficiency

Patient and Complaint: A 40-year-old female presents at the clinic with cough with copious sputum, oppression of the chest, and shortness of breath.

Interrogation: She reports having had this condition for more than 10 years. Two years ago, she suffered from "pneumonia." Furthermore, all symptoms have gradually become more severe. Frequent occurrences of oppression of the chest and difficult respiration are aggravated in winter, early morning, or after exercising, and are combined with palpitations. This has previously been diagnosed as "chronic bronchitis," "pulmonary emphysema," and "slight pulmonary heart disease." She also reports that she suffers from poor appetite and alternating dry and loose stools.

Inspection: Very thin physique, pale face, pale tongue with white coating.

Palpation and Pulse Examination: Deep thin and choppy pulse.

Auscultation and Olfaction: No indications detected.

Pattern Identification: Deficiency of both lung qi and spleen qi.

Explanation: Cough with copious sputum, oppression of the chest and shortness of breath are caused by insufficient lung qi leading to poor dispersing function of the lung. Poor appetite and loose stools are brought about by insufficient spleen qi leading to dysfunction of the spleen in transportation and transformation. Palpitations and pale face and tongue are caused by qi deficiency leading to a poor promotion of blood circulation.

Diagnostic Disease Name: Cough.

7. Lung Qi-Kidney Qi Deficiency

Patient and Complaint: A 31-year-old female presents at the clinic with asthma and shortness of breath marked by prolonged expiration and shortened inspiration.

Interrogation: She reports having had "bronchial asthma" when she was very young. The asthma became more severe eight years ago and has since become chronic. It is accompanied by lassitude and somnolence which is followed by oppression of the chest, asthma, restlessness, general profuse sweating, shortness of breath, occasional urinary incontinence, aversion to wind and cold, palpitation relieved by pressure, dry stools, and scant dark urine.

Inspection: Scaly and dark facial complexion, thin physique.

Pulse Feeling: Deep thin and rapid pulse.

Auscultation and Olfaction: Asthma with prolonged exhalations and shortened inhalations in a low weak voice.

Pattern Identification: Lung qi-kidney qi deficiency pattern.

Explanation: Asthma in low voice, shortness of breath, profuse sweating, and aversion to wind and cold are caused by insufficient lung qi leading to poor promotion of sound production. Urinary incontinence, lassitude, and dark facial complexion are brought about by insufficient kidney qi leading to poor consolidation.

Diagnostic Disease Name: Asthma.

8. Heart Blood-Liver Blood Deficiency

Patient and Complaint: A 47-year-old female presents at the clinic with complaints of palpitations and forgetfulness with insomnia.

Interrogation: She reports having had this condition for three years. It has previously been diagnosed as "menopausal pattern" for which the prescribed treatment has been ineffective. She complains that the symptoms have become more severe. She also reports dream-disturbed sleep, dizziness, tinnitus, dry sensation in both eyes with blurred vision, aching and numbness of the extremities, and scant menstruation.

Inspection: Sallow facial complexion, pale nails, pale tongue with white coating.

Palpation and Pulse Examination: Thin pulse.

Auscultation and Olfaction: No indications detected.

Pattern Identification: Heart blood-liver blood deficiency pattern.

Explanation: Palpitations, insomnia, dream-disturbed sleep, forgetfulness, dizziness, and tinnitus are caused by insufficient heart blood leading to poor nourishment of the heart. Discomfort of the eyes, blurred vision, pale face and nails, decrease of menstruation, and numbness of the body and limbs are brought about by insufficient liver blood leading to poor nourishment of the eyes, tendons, and vessels. Pale tongue and thin pulse are due to poor filling of the blood vessels.

Diagnostic Disease Name: Palpitations and forgetfulness with insomnia.

9. Heart Blood- Spleen Qi Deficiency

Patient and Complaint: A 50-year-old male presents at the clinic with insomnia and palpitations.

Interrogation: He reports having had this condition, which has previously been diagnosed as "chronic coronary heart disease", for three years. He also reports oppression of the chest, lassitude, listlessness, poor appetite, abdominal distension, and occasional loose stools.

Inspection: Pale and puffy face and limbs.

Palpation and Pulse Examination: Thin pulse.

Auscultation and Olfaction: No indications detected.

Pattern Identification: Heart blood-spleen qi deficiency pattern.

Explanation: Pale face, oppression of the chest, insomnia, palpitations, and thin pulse are caused by heart blood deficiency leading to poor nourishment. Poor appetite, loose stools, and abdominal distension are due to spleen qi deficiency leading to poor promotion of digestion. Lassitude and listlessness are brought about by spleen qi deficiency leading to poor promotion of the spirit.

Diagnostic Disease Name: Insomnia.

10. Liver Yin-Kidney Yin Deficiency

Patient and Complaint: A 24-year-old male presents at the clinic with headaches, dizziness, insomnia, and dream-disturbed sleep.

Interrogation: He reports having had this condition, which has previously been diagnosed as "neurasthenia," for half a year. He also reports sleeping only three to four hours per night, with possible sleeplessness all night, forgetfulness, frequent tinnitus, blurred vision, palpitations, irritability, discomfort of the hypochondrium, and poor appetite.

Inspection: Yellow tongue coating.

Palpation and Pulse Examination: Wiry thin and rapid pulse.

Auscultation and Olfaction: No indications detected.

Pattern Identification: Liver yang rising pattern.

Explanation: Blurred vision and discomfort of the hypochondrium are caused by insufficient liver yin leading to poor nourishment; headache, tinnitus, dream-disturbed sleep, irritability, and palpitations are brought about by liver yang rising; forgetfulness and dizziness are due to insufficient kidney yin leading to poor nourishment of the mind.

Diagnostic Disease Name: Insomnia.

11. Lung Yin-Kidney Yin Deficiency

Patient and Complaint: A 64-year-old male presents at the clinic with recurring dry cough, or cough with little sputum retaining blood, and five-palm heat over a period of ten years.

Interrogation: He reports suffering from a dry cough with scant sputum and sometimes hemoptysis, dry throat and nose, and weight loss for the past two years. This was previously diagnosed as "pulmonary tuberculosis." He also complains of soreness and weakness of the lumbar area and limbs, nocturnal emissions, night fever, night sweats, and five-palm heat in recent months.

Inspection: Red zygomatic region, red tongue with scant coating.

Palpation and Pulse Examination: Dry skin with feverish palms and soles, thin rapid pulse.

Auscultation and Olfaction: No indications detected.

Laboratory examination: X-rays show tuberculosis of the lung with cavitation, tubercular fibrosis and perifocal inflammation.

Pattern Identification: Lung yin-kidney yin deficiency pattern.

Explanation: Dry cough, dry throat and nose, hemoptysis and dry skin are due to lung yin deficiency leading to poor nourishment of the lung openings. Scant sputum retaining blood is brought about by deficiency fire damaging the lung network vessels. Chronic illness and soreness and weakness of the lumbar area and knees are caused by insufficiency of kidney yin leading to poor nourishment of tendons and bones. Nocturnal emissions are due to insufficiency of the kidney yin leading to stirring of ministerial fire. Red zygomatic region, five-palm heat, red tongue with scant coating and thin rapid pulse are due to deficiency heat accumulating in the interior of the body.

Diagnostic Disease Name: Consumption.

12. Noninteraction of Heart and Kidney

Patient and Complaint: A 48-year-old male presents at the clinic with insomnia, dream-disturbed sleep, headache, and feeling of distension of the head.

Interrogation: He reports having had this condition for three years, with occasional sleepless nights, restlessness, five-palm heat, tinnitus, and palpitations. He also reports having soreness and pain of the lumbar area and lower limbs, as well as night sweats.

Inspection: Obesity, red cheeks, red tongue with white coating.

Palpation and Pulse Examination: Deep forceless pulse.

Auscultation and Olfaction: No indications detected.

Pattern Identification: Noninteraction between the heart and kidney.

Explanation: Soreness and pain of the lumbar area and limbs, tinnitus, night sweats, and deep weak pulse are caused by deficiency of kidney yin in the lower body leading to poor nourishment; headache with distended feeling, insomnia, dream-disturbed sleep, irritability, and palpitations are brought about by failure of kidney yin to control upward stirring of heart fire affecting the mind.

Diagnostic Disease Name: Insomnia.

13. Spleen Yang-Kidney Yang Deficiency

Patient and Complaint: A 62-year-old male presents at the clinic complaining of diarrhea before dawn and edema.

Interrogation: He reports having had this condition, which has previously been diagnosed as "chronic nephritis," for three months. He also reports that abdominal distension and borborygmus are always followed by diarrhea. He complains of poor appetite, frequent belching, scant and light-colored urine, frequent night urination, lassitude and listlessness, aversion to cold, dizziness, tinnitus, and mild soreness and pain which is constantly occurring in the lumbar area.

Inspection: Pale face; edema of the face, eyelids, and limbs, particularly in the lower limbs.

Palpation and Pulse Examination: Deep thin pulse.

Auscultation and Olfaction: No indications detected.

Laboratory Examination: Urinary protein (+++) with a few granular casts, pus cells and WBC; BUN in blood 40.5 mg/dl; phenol red test 50%; RBC 4,200,000/mm³.

Pattern Identification: Deficiency of both spleen yang and kidney yang.

Explanation: Diarrhea is caused by insufficient kidney yang leading to the life gate fire failing to generate spleen-earth. Abdominal distension, borborygmus, poor appetite, and frequent belching are brought about by insufficient spleen yang leading to dysfunction in transportation and transformation. Abnormal urination, dizziness, tinnitus, aching of the lumbar area, and lassitude and listlessness are due to a deficiency of kidney yang leading to poor promotion of kidney qi, which leads to poor restoration and consolidation of the urinary system. Edema is caused by yang deficiency leading to failure to control the water passage; pale face is caused by poor warmth due to yang deficiency. Deep thin pulse is caused by poor promotion of yang qi.

Diagnostic Disease Name: Diarrhea before dawn.

14. Disharmony between the Liver and Spleen

Patient and Complaint: A 36-year-old female presents at the clinic with complaints of loose stools four to five times per day.

Interrogation: She reports having had this condition for two years and was previously diagnosed as having "chronic colitis" for which the prescribed treatment was ineffective. She states that the symptoms have become more severe in the past month with loose stools occurring four to five times a day. The desire to defecate is always accompanied by severe abdominal pain which is relieved after defecation. She also reports suffering from poor appetite, abdominal distension, borborygmus with intestinal flatus, pain of the hypochondrium, frequent sighing, frequent irritability, scant urine, and discomfort of the anus during defecation.

Inspection: Upon examination, patient was found to have white thick mucosa with the stool and a yellow thin greasy tongue coating.

Palpation and Pulse Examination: Wiry pulse.

Auscultation and Olfaction: No indications detected.

Pattern Identification: Disharmony between the liver and spleen.

Explanation: Abdominal distension, borborygmus, frequent sighing, painful hypochondrium, irritability, and wiry pulse are brought about by stagnation of liver qi. Diarrhea followed by abdominal pain and discomfort of the anus during defecation are caused by obstruction of qi flow in the large intestine. Poor appetite and greasy tongue coating are due to dysfunction of the spleen in transportation and transformation. Dysfunction of the spleen in transportation and transformation is due to stagnation of liver qi attacking the spleen.

Diagnostic Disease Name: Diarrhea.

Bibliography

Wiseman, Nigel and Feng Ye. *A Practical Dictionary of Chinese Medicine. 2nd Edition.* Brookline, MA and Taos, NM. Paradigm Publications, 1998.

Zhu Wenfeng, Chief Editor. *TCM Diagnosis.* TCM Text Book (Higher Education). Shanghai Science and Technology Press, 1995.

Explanation of Terms

Most students of Chinese medicine are aware from the beginning of their studies that no exact relationship exists between a Chinese term and the English language equivalents used in English language textbooks and courses. The Chinese concepts often imply nuances that the English terms may not. There are overlaps and some terms are used for different concepts in different texts. Further, the Chinese terminology of diagnostics is much larger than any of the glossaries applied in the majority of English language texts.

This particular text is meant as a study guide and reference for students and practitioners. Thus the author has chosen a nomenclature and terminology that is as familiar to English-speaking readers as is possible.

Much of the English terminology used in this text can be referenced in *A Practical Dictionary of Chinese Medicine* (Paradigm Publications, 1998). However, to keep the terms familiar to students preparing for their examinations, it has been necessary for some concepts to be presented in a general or more familiar sense rather than with the precise one-to-one correspondence of Chinese concept and English term found in the *Practical Dictionary*. For example, "fever" is used in the present text where the *Practical Dictionary* references "heat pattern," which includes conditions other than measurable fevers. Words such as "accumulation," "dysfunction," "impairment," "insufficiency," convey the general sense of more specific terms such as "gathering," "blockage," "flooding," "reversal," or other terms that indicate the influence of a wide variety of factors including qi, blood, phlegm, cold, heat, wind, emotions, and damages.

With a modicum of diligence and curiosity, readers wishing to obtain the original Chinese or Pinyin from which this present text's terms derive may do so by checking the *Practical Dictionary*. (Descriptives of disease patterns, for instance, may be found under "disease" as well as under individual organ discussions.) Readers who consult the *Practical Dictionary* will be further rewarded with a generous sampling of the nuances of China's venerable medical art. The progressing student will often find that there are a plethora of exact disease configurations attributable to specific pathomechanisms, and that distinguishing them is the triumph and the art of TCM.

Index of Patterns and Pathologies

207, 218-219, 221, 223, 225-227, 233-234, 249, 253, 255, 257-259

ascites, 35-36, 82

ascitic fluids, tumor, or fetus causing qi and blood stagnation, 35

asthma with difficult inhalation, 17, 216

asthma with sputum, 17, 34, 171, 216

asthma, 29, 35, 54-55, 75, 80, 155, 163, 170, 173-176, 219, 221-222, 252-254

attack of external toxic heat or accumulation of damp heat in the skin, 40

attack of external wind accompanied by deep-seated phlegm, 57

attack of pathogens, 52

auricular skin dry and dark, 28

aversion to cold, 64, 68, 80, 88, 93, 95, 97, 134-135, 137, 155, 174, 176, 178, 182, 192, 196, 198, 213, 217, 219, 234, 257

aversion to heat, 144, 146, 155, 157

aversion to wind, 63, 67, 171, 230

aversion to wind and cold, 253-254

B

bad breath, 32, 76, 60-61, 90-91, 188, 251

bedwetting, 96-97, 215-217, 220, 222

behavior, offensive, 190, 196

Bei Ji Qian Jin Yao Fang (Thousand Gold Pieces Prescriptions for Every Emergency), 2

belching, 51, 59-60, 81, 91, 158, 163, 186, 189, 226, 257-258

Bell's palsy, 23, 25, 31, 49

bin lang (semen arecae catechu), 45

bin bing, 236

Bin Hu Mai Jue (Pulse Studies of Bin Hu), 2

bitter taste in mouth, 58, 66, 81, 85-86, 91, 102, 137, 204, 207, 210, 211, 233

bladder cancer, 94

bladder damp heat, 94-95, 217

bleeding in various locations, 166

bleeding pattern, 115, 157

bleeding, 117, 166, 180, 184, 223, 241-242

bleeding, all kinds of chronic, 181

bleeding, dark red and thick, 166

bleeding, heavy, 166

bleeding, light red and thin, 166

bleeding, nasal, 170

bleeding, nose and gum, 157

bleeding, red, thick, and sticky, 166

bleeding→qi collapse→yang exhaustion pattern, 167

blepharitis, 24

blisters like millet seeds, 39

blisters, 207

blockage of blood circulation, 15-16, 43, 48, 190, 194-195

blockage of blood vessels leading to stagnation of the flow of blood, 100

blockage of latent qi, 200

blockage of toxic heat leading to obstruction of blood circulation, 40

blood clots, 71

blood clots obstructing the flow of qi, 71

blood deficiency combined with liver qi stagnation, 119

blood deficiency leading to poor nourishment, 207

blood deficiency, leading to poor nourishment of the lips, 30

blood deficiency leading to poor production of qi, 167

blood deficiency pattern, 14, 21, 30, 40, 32, 48, 73-74, 98, 100, 104, 116-117, 119-120, 164, 209

blood heat pattern, 21, 98, 104, 165-166

blood leaking out of the blood vessels, 164

blood level pattern, 87, 241

blood stagnating in the channels and network vessels, 71

blood stagnating in the chong and ren channels, 73, 99

blood stagnating in the interior of the body leading to failure in the distribution of body fluids, 89

blood stagnating in the vessels, 15-16

blood stasis and blood deficiency pattern, 39

blood stasis in the stomach, 189

blood stasis or deficiency of kidney yang leading to poor opening and closing of the bladder, 212

blood stasis or severe impairment of yin fluids leading to poor nourishment of the skin, 122

blood stasis pattern, 5, 15-16, 30, 37, 48, 71-73, 79, 89, 99-100, 104, 117, 119, 122, 125, 164-165, 166, 194, 198, 200

blood, expectoration of, 157, 163

bloodshot eyes, 85, 144, 204-205, 208, 226

bloody sputum, 226

bloody urine, 217

blurred vision, 100, 202-204, 206-207, 220, 222, 254-256

blurred vision with floaters, 74, 100

body convulsions, 243

body fluid loss leading to sudden vital qi consumption, 115

body fluids accumulating in the abdomen, 82

body fluids collapse pattern, 115

body fluids deficiency pattern, 117

body fluids in massive amounts excreted from the large intestine with stools, 199

body fluids pressing outwards, 232

body fluids producing phlegm when coming together, 172

body fluids retained in the interior of the body, 122

body fluids retained in the skin, 182

body fluids retention pattern, 119

body fluids, sudden loss of, 68

body fluids unimpaired, 135, 182

boil, 40, 158

borborygmus, 199, 257-259

bowels, collapse of, 177

breast tumors, 35

breathing with difficulty, 163

breathing, 51

breathing, shallow and difficult, 171

breathing, weak, 192

brittle nails, 220

bronchial asthma, 253

bronchitis, 252-253

Diagnosis in Traditional Chinese Medicine

bruises, 164
bruising, 219
bulbar conjunctiva and sclera (qi wheel), 25

C

calculi obstructing flow of qi, 71
cancer of the reproductive system, 100-101
cancers, 27, 164
canthus (blood wheel), 25
carbon monoxide poisoning, 30
carbuncle, yang-type, 40
carbuncle, yin-type, 40
carbuncles, 158
cardiac pain, 192, 198, 219
carotid pulsation, 34
cataract, 27
central qi fall leading to poor consolidation of the internal organs, 249
cerebrovascular accident, 18
Chao Yuanfang, 2
cheeks, pigmented, 213
chest distension, 74
chest pain, 61, 174
chest sweating, 70
chest, fullness and oppression in, 175
chicken pox, 123, 158
chills and fever, 78, 172, 242
chills and fever, alternating attacks of, 136
chills and mild fever, 29
chills greater than fever, 64, 68
chills occurring as pathogens enter, 136
chills occurring in windy environment, 64
chills, 50, 63, 104, 137, 151, 154-156, 160, 172-173, 175-176, 230-231, 239, 245
chills, no sweating, 33
cholecystitis, 76
Chong Yang (ST-42), 110
chronic disorders of the nose, 52
chuan jing, 236
Chunyu Yi, 2
Ci Liao (BL-32), 126
clenched teeth and fists, 243
cold accumulating in the chong and ren channels, 100-101
cold accumulating in the interior of the body, 88
cold accumulating in the lower body, 235
cold accumulating in the skin, 122
cold accumulating in the uterus, 212
cold accumulation leading to qi stagnation in the small intestine, 201
cold accumulation pattern, 194, 198
cold attacking the body, 130
cold attacking the exterior of the body, 230
cold attacking the stomach, 188
cold attacking the stomach leading to reversal of stomach qi, 59-60
cold causing the blood vessels to contract, bringing about stagnation of qi and blood, 188
cold congealing in the blood vessels, 43
cold damp, 47, 77, 101

cold damp accumulating in the body, 182, 234
cold damp accumulating in the middle burner lead-ing to poor digestion, 227
cold damp accumulating in the spleen, 183, 185
cold damp accumulating in the spleen leading to poor transportation and transformation, 227
cold damp accumulating in the spleen and stomach lead-ing to bile penetrating into the skin, 39
cold damp accumulating in the stomach leading to rever-sal of stomach qi, 227
cold damp attacking the lower back leading to ob-struction of qi and blood, 37
cold damp disturbing both the spleen and stomach, 26
cold damp disturbing the drainage of bile, 227
cold damp impediment pattern, 37
cold damp leading to obstructed qi and blood circu-lation, 183
cold directly attacking the inside of the body, 138
cold entering and accumulating in the internal or-gans, channels, and network vessels, 72
cold impediment pattern, 37, 78
cold in the lower area of the body, 152
cold invading the internal organs and damaging yang qi, 64
cold limbs, 18, 63-64, 68-69, 80, 87-88, 92-93, 97, 134, 137, 147, 155, 160, 174, 178, 182, 192, 196-198, 213, 217, 219, 234-235, 246
cold limbs relieved by warmth, 135
cold limbs with preference for warmth, 176
cold pattern, 43, 88, 113, 120, 130
cold sensation, 225
cold sensation throughout the body, 185
cold suppressing yang qi, 137
cold sweat, 80, 147, 192, 197
cold sweating on the forehead, 69
cold sweats and cold limbs, 75
cold with false heat manifestations, 150
cold, aversion to, 132
cold, without damage to the body fluids, 137
coldness tending to contract the blood vessels, 208
colic pain in the cardiac region, 192
colic, 200
colitis, 258
collapse of essence and qi of the internal organs, 34
collapse of heart qi or blood, 118
collapse of heart yang, 192, 197
collapse of heart yang leading to blockage of the heart vessel, 75
collapse of heart yang leading to sudden decline of warmth and promotion of the heart, 80
collapse of kidney qi, 96
collapse of life gate fire, 119
collapse of lung qi which fails to support breathing, 35
collapse of qi and yin, 21
collapse of stomach qi, 59, 118
collapse of vital qi, 118
collapse of vital qi leading to poor nourishment and promotion of the mind, 53
collapse of yang, 115
collapse of yang qi, 69, 124

collapse of yang qi leading to poor consolidation of body fluids, 69
collapse of yang qi leading to poor warmth of the whole body and limbs, 192
collapse of yin, 115
collapsed yang qi flowing outwards, 118
collapsed yin fluids flowing outward, 69
color blindness, 202-203, 220, 222
coma and delirium, 50
common cold, 251
complexion, abnormal colorations of, 13
complexion, blue-green, 15
complexion, pale black, blue-green
complexion, black
complexion, black scaly dry
complexion, black haggard
complexion, black puffy
complexion, dim, sallow, or pale, 220
complexion, lifeless, 12
complexion, normal, 12-13
complexion, pale or sallow, 165
complexion, pale white, 14
complexion, red, 14
complexion, sallow, 20-21, 164, 180-181, 184
complexion, vigorous, 12
complexion, white, 13
complexion, yellow, 14
congealed blood stagnating in the abdomen, 125
congenital defect from kidney essence deficiency, 38
conjunctivitis, 25
consciousness, sudden loss of, 163
constipation without flatus, 200
constipation, 50, 58, 65, 70, 76, 90, 92, 95, 99, 104, 135, 144, 157, 165, 177, 188, 194, 232, 246
constitution, weak, 16
constitutional insufficiency of body fluids leading to poor lubrication of the intestinal tract, 177
constitutional yang deficiency leading to poor warmth of the body surface, 64, 138
constitutional yin deficiency, 141
constriction of the blood vessels by accumulated cold leading to obstructed blood circulation, 165
constriction of the liver channel due to excess cold, 202
consumption from a chronic illness leading to kid-ney yang and yin deficiency, 39
consumption of body fluids due to heat, 56
consumption of body fluids leading to a poor source for urine, 95
consumption of raw, cold, or unclean food or drinks causing obstruction of spleen and stomach qi, lead-ing to poor promotion of digestion, 156
consumption of yang qi leading to poor warmth, 138
consumption of yin fluids producing deficiency heat, 141
consumption, 256
contraction of blood vessels, 16
contraction of blood vessels leading to poor filling and nourishing of blood, 135
convulsions and spasms of the limbs, 19, 209
convulsions of the body, 206, 241

convulsions of the extremities, 197, 202
convulsions or tremors of the fingers and toes, 242
coronary heart disease, 255
cough and asthma, 17, 245
cough and asthma, paroxysmal, 226
cough with clear thin sputum, 176
cough with copious sputum, 252-253
cough with little sputum retaining blood, 256
cough with low voice, 252
cough with scant and sticky sputum, 157, 218
cough with sputum, 52
cough with thick and sticky sputum, 159
cough with weak voice, 170
cough, 17, 29, 34, 56-57, 132, 154-155, 160, 163, 170-176, 219, 221-222, 239, 245, 250-253, 256
cough, dry, 171, 218
cough, dry with scant sputum, 256
cough, dry with sticky and scant sputum, 173
cough, severe after exercising, 170
coughing blood, 170-171, 173, 218, 226
coughing, 51, 55, 75, 80, 151
crying and laughing, 196
cun kou, 107-108, 111
cupping, 3

D

Da Chang Shu (BL-25), 126
Da Ling (PC-7), 125
damage to yin fluids, 16
damp accumulating in the interior of the body, 88
damp accumulating in the spleen leading to dys-function in transportation and transformation, 185
damp accumulation pattern, 14
damp and phlegm pattern, 176
damp disturbance in the spleen leading to poor transpor-tation and transformation, 89
damp disturbing the joints leading to stagnation of qi and blood, 38
damp disturbing the spleen, 89
damp heat accumulating in the bladder, 217
damp heat accumulating in the body, 178, 217
damp heat accumulating in the gallbladder channel and struggling against vital qi, 211
damp heat accumulating in the interior of the body, 89, 247
damp heat accumulating in the intestinal tract and dis-turbing the flow of qi, 93
damp heat accumulating in the intestinal tract and im-pairing the blood vessels of the large intes-tine, 177
damp heat accumulating in the large intestine, 93, 178
damp heat accumulating in the liver and gallblad-der, 26, 75
damp heat accumulating in the liver and gallbladder channels leading to bile penetrating the skin, 39, 207
damp heat accumulating in the liver and gallbladder leading to dysfunction of the liver and gall-bladder in dispersing and descending, 227
damp heat accumulating in the liver and gallbladder leading to stagnation of liver qi, 81

damp heat accumulating in the lower burner, 94-95

damp heat accumulating in the middle burner and steaming upward, 69

damp heat accumulating in the middle burner lead-ing to spleen and stomach qi stagnation, 247

damp heat accumulating in the spleen, 24, 183, 185

damp heat accumulating in the spleen and stomach, 30-31

damp heat accumulating in the stomach and intes-tines leading to impairment of qi and blood, 58

damp heat accumulating in the stomach and spleen and steaming upward, 91

damp heat disturbing the drainage of bile, 227

damp heat disturbing the flow of liver qi, 227

damp heat disturbing the flow of stomach qi, 227

damp heat disturbing the intestinal tract and damag-ing the blood vessels, 93

damp heat disturbing the large intestine leading to qi stagnation, 93

damp heat from both the liver and gallbladder, 227

damp heat obstructing channel and collateral qi, 247

damp heat pattern, 24, 30-31, 47, 58, 61, 69, 70, 89-90, 101

damp heat retained in the body, 184

damp heat stagnating in the body, 211

damp heat steaming bile outward, 207

damp heat steaming outward, 61, 70

damp heat steaming the gallbladder, leading to an out-flow of bile, 184

damp heat steaming upward, 207

damp impediment pattern, 38, 72, 78, 156

damp invading and retained in the joint leading to stag-nation of qi and blood, 78

damp obstructing the flow of qi and blood, 72

damp pattern, 5, 46-47, 88, 115-117, 120, 122

damp phlegm accumulating in the lung leading to lung qi stagnation, 56

damp phlegm obstructing the lung, 175-176

damp phlegm or blood stasis obstructing the chan-nels and network vessels, 83

damp phlegm pattern, 56

damp retention pattern, 95

damp warm pattern, 39, 65

damp warm retained in the interior of the body, 66

dampness attacking the interior, 156

Dan Shu (BL-19), 126

dandruff, 21

deafness, 84, 204, 223-224

decline of essence and qi of the internal organs, 36-37

decline of fire from the life gate leading to poor warmth, 97

decline of fire in the life gate leading to poor con-solidation, 135

decline of kidney qi, 216

decline of kidney qi leading to poor consolidation, 61

decline of kidney qi leading to poor consolidation of the bladder, 96

decline of life gate fire brought on by a deficiency of kidney yang, 212

decline of life gate fire leading to poor consolida-tion of semen, 213

decline of life gate fire leading to poor warmth, 96

decline of life gate fire leading to poor warmth of the spleen, 212-213

decline of vital qi, 29-30

decline of vital qi leading to separation of yin and yang, 52

declining yang floating upward, 69

declining yang qi flowing outwards, 114

deep-seated heat in the yang ming bowel, 232

defecation with discomfort of the anus, 226

defecation, difficult, 92, 179

deficiency and cold pattern, 13

deficiency cold accumulating in the body, 178, 187, 199

deficiency cold accumulating in the large intestine lead-ing to poor warmth of the abdomen, 177

deficiency cold accumulating in the small intestine lead-ing to poor warmth of the abdomen, 199

deficiency cold of the stomach leading to poor warmth of the abdomen, 186

deficiency cold pattern, 14, 49, 58, 64, 72, 91, 95, 115, 119, 123-124, 133

deficiency ejaculation for men

deficiency fire accumulating in the body, 171, 214

deficiency fire compressing blood out of the ves-sels, 214

deficiency fire compressing body fluids outward, 193

deficiency fire damaging the lung collateral chan-nels, 171

deficiency fire damaging the lung network vessels, 256

deficiency fire flaring up and consuming body flu-ids, 187, 214

deficiency fire flaring upward, 28

deficiency fire impairing the body fluids, 171

deficiency fire spreading all over the body, 193

deficiency fire steaming outward, 171

deficiency heat, 179

deficiency heat accumulating in the body, 134, 204-206, 235, 256

deficiency heat accumulating in the stomach leading to its inability to regulate stomach qi, 186

deficiency heat consuming body fluids, 247

deficiency heat pattern, 26-28, 30, 48-49, 72, 115, 123, 133, 150

deficiency heat steaming body fluids outward, 235

deficiency liver wind, 242

deficiency of both lung qi and spleen qi, 253

deficiency of both qi and blood, 49

deficiency of both spleen and kidney qi, 25

deficiency of both spleen yang and kidney yang, 258

deficiency of heart qi or heart blood, 118

deficiency of heart yang, 15

deficiency of kidney essence, 212

deficiency of kidney yang, 16

deficiency of kidney yang leading to dysfunction of the bladder, 212

deficiency of kidney yang leading to poor promo-tion of kidney qi, 258

deficiency of kidney yin in the lower body leading to poor nourishment, 257
deficiency of kidney yin leading to the rising of ministerial fire, 212
deficiency of liver and kidney yin in the lower body, 205
deficiency of lung and spleen yang leading to poor promotion of lung qi, 57
deficiency of lung yin combined with deficiency of kidney yin, 224
deficiency of qi, blood, and yang leading to poor nourishment and circulation of blood, 50
deficiency of qi, blood, yin, and yang bringing about poor warmth and nourishment of the body, 78
deficiency of spleen and kidney yang, 22
deficiency of spleen and stomach qi, 20
deficiency of spleen qi, 40
deficiency of spleen qi leading to dysfunction of the spleen in transportation, 182
deficiency of spleen qi leading to inability to consolidate the internal organs, 162
deficiency of spleen qi providing a poor source for qi and blood, 86
deficiency of stomach yin, 186
deficiency of yang qi leading to poor warmth, 124
deficiency pattern, 13, 19, 21, 43, 49-54, 56-59, 71-73, 77-78, 82-84, 92, 94, 122, 124, 130
delayed development, 35
delirium with high voice, 190
delirium, 49, 87, 134, 144, 155, 240- 242, 246
depression of gallbladder qi, 211
depression, 162, 197
depressive psychosis, 159, 197
desire for hot drinks, 147
desire to lie down, 137
desire to speak, 53
desquamation, 156
deviation of the eyes and mouth, 205, 209
diabetes, 61, 88, 95
diarrhea alternating with dry stools, 93
diarrhea at dawn, 177
diarrhea before dawn, 213, 257-258
diarrhea followed by abdominal pain, 93
diarrhea with pain and discomfort of the anus dur-ing defecation, 259
diarrhea with partially digested fat in the stools, 93
diarrhea with white turbid liquid, 58
diarrhea, 21, 68, 88-89, 93, 155-156, 160, 178, 185, 215, 219, 220, 222, 234-235, 249, 257-259
difficulty falling asleep, 86
diphtheria, 33, 35, 158
discomfort and fullness of the upper abdomen, 69-70
discomfort of the anus after defecation, 250
discomfort of the chest, hypochondrium, breasts, and lower abdomen, 202
discomfort of the hypochondrium, 255
disharmony between liver and spleen, 93, 258
disharmony between liver and stomach, 91, 226
disorder occurring in the blood system that does not involve bladder qi, 231
distending pain in the head, 71

distending pain occurring in the chest, hypochon-drium, and abdominal region, 163
distending pain occurring in the chest, upper and lower abdomen, 71
distending pain of the abdomen, 90
distending pain of the chest, hypochondrium, breasts, and lower abdomen, 202
distending pain of the head, 208
distending pain of the hypochondrium, 227
distending pain of the lower abdomen, 94
distension and discomfort of the hypochondrium, 81
distension and fullness of the abdomen, 93
distension and fullness of the hypochondrium, 226
distension and fullness of the upper abdomen, 159-160, 183, 187, 207, 227
distension and pain in the hypochondrium, 210
distension and pain of the chest and hypochon-drium, 226
distension and pain of the upper abdomen, 156
distension around the breasts, 99
distension of the abdomen, 82, 89, 91- 92, 102, 160, 184
distension of the eyeballs, 27
distension of the head, 257
distension of the hypochondrium, 58, 81
distension of the upper abdomen, 59, 91
distension or pain, 144
distension under the right hypochondrium, 250
disturbance by damp and retention of body fluids, 46
disturbance by damp phlegm, 47
disturbance of blood, 42
disturbance of spleen yang and spleen qi leading to poor transportation and transformation, 135
dizziness and tinnitus, 102-103
dizziness with pale complexion, 79
dizziness with stabbing pain of the head following trauma, 79
dizziness, 21, 32, 34, 66, 79, 85, 87, 89, 97-98, 100, 102-103, 137, 162-164, 191, 193, 202-206, 209-210, 214, 219-222, 233, 249, 252, 254-258
downbearing pain in the lower abdomen, 103
downbearing sensation in the abdomen., 249
downward flow of cold damp, 182-183, 227
downward flow of damp heat, 183, 199, 211, 216
downward flow of damp heat along the liver chan-nel, 207
downward flow of damp heat from the large intes-tine, 93
downward flow of damp heat into the lower burner, 217
downward flow of excess heat, 61
downward flow of liver and gallbladder damp heat, 61
downward flow of turbid qi, 189
downward flow of undigested food to the large intestine, 180, 199
dream-disturbed sleep, 70, 86, 97, 218, 224, 254-257
dribbling urination, 95
drink, no desire for, 182, 187
drooling with clear saliva, 187-188
drooling with foamy saliva, 197
drooling with yellow sticky saliva, 31
drooling, 89, 205

Diagnosis in Traditional Chinese Medicine

drowsiness, 190

drug, food, or alcohol poisoning, 19, 27, 49, 158

dry cracked lips, 246

dry mouth, 137, 179, 204

dry mouth and lips, 218

dry mouth and throat, 70, 171, 176, 187, 214, 247

dry skin, 68, 256

dry stools, 30, 92, 151, 174, 184, 204, 209, 253

dry throat, 233

dryness and discomfort of the eyeball, 85

dryness and discomfort of the eyes, 206, 218

dryness and heat impairing body fluids, 30

dryness attacking the exterior, 156

dryness attacking the lung, 157, 173, 176

dryness invading the exterior of the body, 156

dryness pattern, 46

dryness remaining in the exterior of the body, 173

Du Qingbi, 2

dull expression, 137

dull pain in the gastric region with preference for warmth and pressure, 187

dull reactions, 190, 197

dysfunction in lifting lucid yang, 234

dysfunction in storing kidney essence, 212

dysfunction of body fluids distribution, 178

dysfunction of wei qi in dispersing, 132

dysfunction of internal organs, 115

dysfunction of metabolism of body fluids, 212

dysfunction of qi and blood of the internal organs, 42

dysfunction of splenic transformation and transportation, 91

dysfunction of the bladder, 217

dysfunction of the bladder in storing urine and di-recting urination, 216

dysfunction of the gallbladder in dispersing and spread-ing, 210

dysfunction of the heart in governing the mind, leading to mental confusion, 190

dysfunction of the heart in governing vitality, 197

dysfunction of the internal organs leading to pro-duction of phlegm, phlegm fluids, water qi, damp, blood stasis, or food stagnation causing obstruction of the flow of qi, 144

dysfunction of the kidney leading to impaired open-ing and closing of the bladder, 148

dysfunction of the large intestine in transmission, 177

dysfunction of the liver in dispersing and precipitat-ing, 201

dysfunction of the liver in dispersing and spreading, 205, 207, 235

dysfunction of the liver in regulating qi flow, 194-195

dysfunction of the liver in spreading and precipitat-ing, 163

dysfunction of the liver in spreading and precipitat-ing, leading to qi stagnating in the liver chan-nel, 202

dysfunction of the liver in storing blood, 202

dysfunction of the lung in dispersing and descend-ing, 163, 170

dysfunction of the lung in dispersing and precipitat-ing qi, 132, 172-175, 239

dysfunction of the lung in draining water down-wards to the bladder, 175

dysfunction of the lung in governing qi and respira-tion, 170

dysfunction of the lung in governing the metabo-lism of the body fluids, 170

dysfunction of the lung in regulating water passage, 175

dysfunction of the lung, spleen, and kidney, 36

dysfunction of the lung, spleen, and kidney leading to abnormal metabolism of body fluids, 95

dysfunction of the metabolism of body fluids, 213

dysfunction of the opening and closing of the blad-der orifice leading to water remaining in the lower burner, 231

dysfunction of the small intestine in separating lucid nutrition from turbid waste, 199

dysfunction of the small intestine in storing and digest-ing, 199

dysfunction of the small intestine in transportation, 200

dysfunction of the spleen and stomach, 211

dysfunction of the spleen in keeping blood circulat-ing inside the blood vessels, 180, 184

dysfunction of the spleen in promoting lucid yang qi, 184

dysfunction of the spleen in transportation and transfor-mation, 180-181, 183-184, 259

dysfunction of the spleen in transporting damp leading to the retention of body fluids, 180

dysfunction of the stomach in precipitating qi lead-ing to reversal of stomach qi, 186

dysfunction of the stomach in regulating and pre-cipitating, 163

dysfunction of the stomach in storage and digestion, 186-187

dysfunction of the thoroughfare and controlling channels in regulating the menses, 202

dysfunction of transportation and transformation, 135

dysfunctional uterine bleeding, 215

dysmenorrhea with dark-colored menstruation, 165

dysmenorrhea, 100, 202, 214

dyspepsia, 81

dysphoria, 151, 209

dysuria, 144

E

ear seeding, 3

Eastern Han, 2

ecchymosis, 29, 32, 99, 104, 164, 241

eczema, 207

edema, 22, 34, 36, 39, 55, 81-82, 95, 160, 170, 175, 180, 182-183, 185, 197, 212-213, 219, 225, 250-251, 257-258

emaciation, 17, 35-37, 89-91, 142, 171, 180-181

emotional depression, 59-60, 81, 91, 93, 99, 190, 226

emotional distress, 18, 21, 82, 96-97, 118

emotional excitement, 190

emphysema, 34

enuresis, 215-216, 219

epilepsy, 54, 159, 197

epistaxis, 241

exterior heat coexisting simultaneously with liver and kidney yin deficiency, 248

exterior heat-interior cold pattern, 151

exterior heat pattern, 29, 38, 47, 52, 63-64, 67, 73, 119, 121, 123, 130-132, 141, 151

exterior pattern, 13, 42, 45, 55-56, 68, 78, 85, 104, 113-114, 122, 129

exterior wind, 154

external cold entering the interior of the body and producing heat, 151

external dampness leading to damp accumulating on the exterior of the body and obstructing qi in the channels and network vessels, 156

external heat stagnating on the surface of the body, 121

external pathogenic wind cold attacking the exterior of the body, 132

external pathogens attacking the exterior of the body, 42, 45, 131, 144

external pathogens attacking the lung, 55, 170

external pathogens attacking the lung leading to obstruction of lung qi, 51

external pathogens entering the interior of the body, 42

external pathogens invading the area of the body that is half exterior and half interior, 233

external pathogens remaining in the exterior of the body, 231

external wind, 21

external wind attacking the exterior of the body leading to looseness of the muscular intersti-ces, 64

external wind attacking the joints leading to stagna-tion of qi and blood, 78

external wind cold attacking and stirring upward, 73

external wind damp attacking and stirring upward, 74

external wind heat attacking and flaring upward, 73-74, 85

external wind invading and inducing internal wind, 50

externally attacking damp heat accumulating on the surface of the body, 39

extravasation of blood, 189

extreme cold accumulating in the three yin chan-nels, 118

extreme deficiency appearing as excess manifesta-tions, 150

extreme excess appearing as deficiency manifesta-tions, 150

extreme heat accompanied by yin deficiency in the ying level, 240

extreme heat accumulating in the three yang chan-nels, 118

extreme heat causing liver wind to rise, 15

extreme heat causing stirring of liver wind, 31

extreme heat engendering wind and stirring upward, 27

extreme heat entering yin and blood levels, 48

extreme heat excessively promoting blood circula-tion, causing extravasation, 241

extreme heat from the lung and stomach accumulat-ing in the throat, 32

extreme heat impairing yin deficiency in the blood level, 241

extreme heat inducing an attack of liver wind, 31, 50, 206, 241

extreme heat leading to the exhaustion of body flu-ids, 47

extreme heat pattern, 209

extreme heat penetrating the pericardium, 52-53

extreme heat steaming outward, 240

extreme impairment of body fluids due to heat, 50

extreme pain, 18

extreme spleen qi deficiency leading to poor promo-tion of the internal organs, 94

extreme summerheat, 155

exuberant heart fire stirring upwards, 194

eyelid (flesh wheel), 24

eyes and mouth, deviation, 23

eyes bloodshot and painful, 27

eyes painful, 26

eyes, bloodshot, 74-75

eyes, discomfort of, 27

eyes, discomfort and dry rough feeling, 223

eyesight, dim, 85

F

face and limbs pale and puffy, 255

face and lips, pale, 21, 74, 84

face and tongue, pale, 68

face suddenly turning pale, 192, 197

face, dusky, 165

face, dusky with pigmented spots, 102

face, flushed, 52, 75, 139

face, pale, 69, 79-80, 103, 135, 137, 158, 164, 171, 191, 193, 203, 206, 249, 253, 255, 257-258

face, pale puffy 134, 219

face, pale with puffy eyelids, 252

face, puffy, 175, 197

face, sallow, dry, or pale, 181

face, sallow or pale, 222

facial complexion, dark, 254

facial complexion, pale, 155

facial complexion, sallow, 254

facial complexion, scaly and dark, 253

facial paralysis, 23

facial swelling, 22

failure of wei qi to warm the exterior of the body, 64

failure of the lung to drain the water passages, 22

failure of the small intestine to separate the food-stuff from the dregs, 199

failure of the spleen and kidney to distribute and drain body fluids, 22

failure to promote blood circulation, 192

fainting, 247

false vitality, 10

febrile diseases, 61, 68

fecal incontinence, 94

Fei Shu (BL 13), 125

fever accompanied by shivering, 211

fever aggravated at night, 240, 242

fever and chills, 35, 76, 211

fever and chills alternating at irregular intervals, 136

fever and chills at alternating at regular intervals, 136

fever greater than chills, 64, 67, 132, 157

fever occurring as the struggle of vital qi and evil qi
waxes, 136

fever, 17, 20, 23, 33, 49-50, 52, 54, 61, 63-65, 67, 73,
85, 88, 92, 95, 98, 104, 133, 144, 151, 155, 157,
172,-173, 175-176, 209, 230-231, 239-242, 245

fever, afternoon, 223, 243

fever, hemorrhagic, 158

fever, high, 65, 69, 87, 139, 174, 206, 232, 243, 246, 248

fever, high with severe sweating, 30

fever, high in children, 31

fever, high, occurring in febrile disease, 18

fever, high with profuse sweating, 146

fever, low-grade, 134, 139, 154-156, 160

fever, mild, 65-66

fever, nocturnal, 204, 206

fever, tidal, 134, 155-156

feverish palms and soles, 256

feverish sensation of the body, 185

fevers, chills, 56

fighting between vital qi and pathogenic factors occurring in the shao yang channel, 211

fighting between vital qi and pathogens occurring in the
exterior of the body, 230

fingers and toes, trembling of, 202, 206, 243

fire accumulating in the stomach, 76

fire attacking the exterior of the body, 157

fire compressing the blood and forcing it out of the
blood vessels, 157

fire damaging the blood vessels of the lung, 170

fire penetrating the pericardium, 157

fire stirring upward, 81

fists and teeth clenched, 30

fists clenched, 31

five kinds of flaccidity in infants, 212

five kinds of retardation and flaccidity, 20-21, 34, 35,
37-38

five kinds of retardation in infants, 212

five leaks, 215

five palm heat, 27

five wheel theory, 23

five-palm fever, 242

five-palm heat, 32, 56, 65-66, 68, 70, 79-80, 85, 89, 123,
134, 139, 142, 171, 176, 187, 193, 197, 204, 206,
214, 218, 223, 235, 247, 256-257

flaccidity of the limbs, 142

flaccidity of the lower limbs, 78

flaccidity, 38, 105

flaring of stomach fire, 60

flaring up of blood heat, 21

flaring up of deficiency fire, 26, 214

flaring up of deficiency or excess heart fire, 190

flaring up of heart fire, 25, 190, 194

flaring up of stomach fire leading to stagnation of qi and
blood, 188

flaring up of the mind, 134

flaring up of wind heat or toxic fire, 23

flatus, 258

floaters, 202-203, 207, 220, 222

fluid retention, 36

flushed face, 85, 95, 144, 157, 204-205, 208, 246

flushed zygomatic area, 187

fontanel, 19, 20

food intake, 10

food intake, improper, 158

food stagnating in the stomach, 189

food stagnation leading to stagnation of stomach qi, 158,
186

food stagnation, 59, 61, 71, 81, 87, 90-91, 93-94, 117,
119-120, 158

foot jue yin, 110

foot shao yang, 28, 33, 209

foot shao yin, 32, 110

foot tai yang, 28, 33

foot tai yin, 110

foot yang ming, 28, 31, 33, 110

forgetfulness, 21, 193, 197, 222-223, 231, 254-256

four diagnostic methods, 6

four greatnesses, 236

fullness and abdominal distension with constipation, 246

fullness and discomfort of the upper abdomen, 81

fullness and distension of the abdomen, 58

fullness and distension of the chest and hypochon-drium,
136

fullness and distension of the chest and upper ab-domen,
247

fullness and distension of the hypochondrium and abdomen, 233

fullness and distension of the upper abdomen, 59, 87,
183

fullness and oppression of the chest, 170

fullness and pain of the upper abdomen, 158

fullness of the abdomen, 234

fullness of the chest, 29, 52, 54-55

fullness of the chest and hypochondrium, 66

fullness of the chest, hypochondrium, breasts, and lower
abdomen, 202

fullness of the upper abdomen, 87, 89, 91, 94, 235

fullness of the upper abdomen and the hypochon-drium,
60

fullness or oppression in the upper abdomen, 185

fullness, distension, accumulation, or pain of the affected area, 144

furuncle, 40, 158

fuzzy thoughts, 196

G

gallbladder channel damp heat, 211

gallbladder depression–phlegm fire stirring upward, 81,
86

gallbladder heat steaming upward, 137

gallbladder impediment pattern, 117

gallbladder qi steaming upward, 204, 233

Gan Shu (BL-18), 126

gangrene of toe, 18

gas rumbling upward (running piglet qi), 235

gasping, 55

German measles, 158

gingivitis, 60

glaucoma, 27

globus hystericus (plum-pit qi), 203
goiter, 33, 159, 203
gradual consumption of yang qi, 147
groaning, 52
Guan Yuan (CV-4), 126
gum bleeding, 60, 76, 90
gums with redness, swelling, and pain, 32
gums with redness, swelling, severe pain, ulcera-tion, 32
gums, pale, 32
gums, recurrent bleeding, 32

H

hair loss, 21
hair, dry without luster, 21
hair, premature graying, 21, 214
hair, tangled sparse and dry, 22
half exterior–half interior pattern, 136
Han Feixia, 2
Han Shi Yi Tong (Han's Comprehensive Medical Views), 2
hand shao yang, 28, 110
hand shao yin, 110
hand tai yang, 28
hand tai yin, 110
hand yang ming, 33, 110
hard masses, 101
he bing, 236
He Gu (LI-4), 110
head, heaviness of, 156
headache occurring in the forehead, 74
headache occurring in the posterior of the head, 74
headache occurring in the temples, 74
headache occurring in the top of the head, 74
headache radiating to the upper back aggravated by wind, 73
headache with a sensation of heaviness of the head, limbs, and the whole body, 74
headache with distended feeling, 257
headache with distending sensation of the head, 74
headache with distension, 204-205
headache with dizziness, 74
headache with hollow sensation, 74
headache, 21, 27, 34, 50, 60, 66, 68, 73, 85, 104, 132, 151, 155, 163, 172, 176, 205, 239, 242, 245, 250-251, 255-257
headache, jue yin, 74
headache, shao yang, 74
headache, sudden, severe, and persistent, 73
headache, tai yang, 74
headache, yang ming, 74
hearing, weak, 242, 247
heart blood deficiency, 80, 193, 220
heart blood deficiency combined with liver blood defi-ciency, 222
heart blood deficiency combined with spleen qi defi-ciency, 223
heart blood deficiency leading to poor nourishment, 255
heart blood–liver blood deficiency pattern, 222, 254
heart blood not circulating smoothly in the heart vessel, 194

heart blood–spleen qi deficiency pattern, 255
heart blood stasis pattern, 74, 80-81
heart dysfunction in promoting blood circulation, 219
heart fire failing to be controlled by kidney yin, 257
heart fire flaring up and stirring the mind, 200, 235
heart fire flaring upward, compressing heart fluids out-wards, 70
heart fire moving down to the small intestine, 200
heart fire rising pattern, 25
heart qi deficiency combined with lung qi defi-ciency, 221
heart qi deficiency leading to blood stasis, 252
heart qi deficiency pattern, 53, 191, 197, 219
heart qi-lung qi deficiency pattern, 220, 252
heart vessel, blockage of, 15
heart vessel obstruction pattern, 197
heart yang collapse, 75, 197
heart yang deficiency, 197, 219
heart yang deficiency combined with kidney yang defi-ciency, 225
heart yang-kidney yang deficiency, 225
heart yang qi deficiency leading to poor promotion of qi and blood in the heart vessel, 74
heart yang qi deficiency pattern, 80
heart yin deficiency combined with kidney yin defi-ciency leading to poor nourishment of the body and deficiency heat, 235
heart yin deficiency pattern, 80, 193, 197, 218
heart-kidney yang deficiency leading to collapse of or-gan function, 87
heart-kidney yang deficiency pattern, 87
heart-spleen deficiency pattern, 70, 86
heat accumulating in the body and forcing blood out of the vessels, 99
heat accumulating in the chest, 17
heat accumulating in the heart and spleen, 49
heat accumulating in the heart, lung, liver, and gall-bladder, 48
heat accumulating in the interior of the body, 43, 48, 121
heat accumulating in the intestinal tract with dry stools, 92
heat accumulating in the lung, 56
heat accumulating in the skin, 122
heat accumulating in the upper part of the body, 235
heat and pain in the breast, 35
heat attacking the body, 130
heat attacking the stomach leading to reversal of stom-ach qi, 59
heat attack, pathogenic, 141
heat causing the body fluids to become concen-trated, 172
heat dispersing outward when yang ming qi is rising, 232
heat entering the blood level, 241
heat impairing body fluids, 139, 240
heat impediment pattern, 38, 78
heat in the blood compressing the blood out of the ves-sels, 98
heat in the blood level accumulating in the body and damaging the uterine network vessels, 104

heat in the limbs, 133
heat in the upper area of the body, 152
heat pattern, 42-43, 48-50, 113, 116, 120-122, 130, 139
heat penetrating the pericardium, 87, 240
heat speeding up blood circulation, 139
heat steaming body fluid outwards, 122
heat stirring in the mind, 137, 241
heat with false cold manifestations, 122, 150
heaviness and pain of the joints, 156
heaviness in the affected limb, 78
heaviness of the body, 54, 88, 156
heaviness of the head, 69-70, 159, 205, 209
heaviness of the head and body, 65, 85, 87, 183, 185, 227, 247
heaviness of the head and lightness of foot, 205
hemafecia, 184
hematemesis, 241
hematochezia, 189, 241
hematopathy, 29, 32
hematuria, 184, 199, 250
hemiparalysis, 50, 69, 205
hemiparesis, 83, 165, 209
hemiplegia, 18, 23
hemophilia, 30
hemoptysis, 165, 256
hemorrhage, subcutaneous, 184
hepatic diseases, 82
hepatitis, 75, 250
hernia, 201
herpes, 30
hiccups, 51, 58-59, 76, 90-91, 163, 186-187, 226
high blood pressure, 250
hoarseness, 52
hot sensation and pain in the affected area, 165
huang lian (rhizoma coptidis), 45
Huang Di Nei Jing (Yellow Emperor's Classic of Internal Medicine), 107
hunger with no desire for food, 76, 186, 235
hydrocephalus, 20, 28
hyperactive stomach receives too much food which a weak spleen is unable to transport and trans-form, 90
hyperactivity of the stomach in storing food and digesting, 188
hyperactivity of the stomach–weakness of the spleen, 90
hypertension, 34
hyperthyroidism, 25, 27
hypochondrium distension, 26
hypochondrium pain, 250
hypofunction in consolidation of stools, urine, se-men; and of the fetus and menses, 220
hypofunction in promotion of blood circulation and the mind, 219
hypofunction in promotion of respiration and voice, 219
hypofunction in transportation and transformation of foodstuff and damp, 219
hypofunction of the internal organs leading to poor in-vigoration of the physical body and the vital-ity, 162
hypoxia, 30

I

impairment of blood vessels, 217
impairment of body fluids, 36, 46, 49, 88, 134, 188, 194, 232, 235
impairment of body fluids leading to poor source for sweat, 68
impairment of body fluids, severe, 21, 39
impairment of both stomach qi and stomach yin, 48
impairment of ying yin, 240
impairment of heart qi leading to poor nourishment of the mind, 53
impairment of kidney essence, 117
impairment of kidney essence and qi, 27
impairment of kidney yin, 16
impairment of kidney yin and yang leading to de-cline of life gate fire causing poor warmth, 96
impairment of kidney yin leading to poor nourish-ment of the teeth, 31
impairment of kidney yin leading to stirring upward of ministerial fire, 97
impairment of lung and kidney leading to lung qi accu-mulating in the chest, 34
impairment of spleen qi leading to failure to raise lucid yang, 249
impairment of stomach qi, 189
impairment of the blood vessels in the lung, 173
impairment of the blood vessels leading to putrefy-ing pustulating flesh, 178
impairment of the lung collateral channels leading to poor circulation of qi and blood, 173
impairment of yang qi leading to yang exhaustion, 147
impairment of yin fluids, 17, 31, 133, 196, 241
impairment of yin fluids leading to yin exhaustion, 146
impediment pattern, 15-16, 18, 117-118, 120
impotence, 96-97, 212-213, 219
improper food intake impairing the spleen and stomach, leading to poor digestion, 81
improper food intake leading to reversal of stomach qi, 87
inability to consolidate the qi of the thoroughfare and controlling channels, 181
inability to govern blood circulating inside the blood vessels, 181
inability to grasp qi, 17
inability to guide qi upward and nourish the tongue, 162
inability to lie down, 55
inability to promote blood circulation, 192
inability to receive air, 216
inability to regulate the flow of stomach qi, 187
inability to soothe liver and gallbladder, 183
inappropriate treatment, 147
inappropriate treatment damaging spleen yang when external heat attacks, 151
inappropriate treatment damaging vital qi, 150
incessant talking, 196
indigestion, 158
infantile convulsions, 15, 19, 25, 27, 30, 42, 50, 123
infantile malnutrition, 22, 105
infantile paralysis, 18

infantile persistent mild fever occurring in summer, 66

infants with the five kinds of retardation and flac-cidity, 34

infertility, 212-213, 215

insecurity of kidney qi, 103

insomnia with dream-disturbed sleep, 193

insomnia, 21, 25, 79, 87, 166, 190, 193-194, 196-197, 210, 214, 218, 222-224, 235, 240, 254-257

instability of gallbladder qi, 210

insufficiency of blood, 21, 32

insufficiency of blood and yin resulting in poor nour-ishment, 71

insufficiency of blood bringing about internal dry-ness and deficiency heat, 104

insufficiency of blood leading to poor nourishment of chong and ren channels, 73, 100

insufficiency of blood leading to poor nourishment of the body and limbs, 220

insufficiency of blood leading to poor nourishment of the head, 74

insufficiency of blood leading to poor nourishment of the tongue, 48

insufficiency of blood leading to poor source of men-struation, 98

insufficiency of body fluids leading to a lack of source for urine, 148

insufficiency of both qi and blood leading to poor nour-ishment and circulation of blood, 49

insufficiency of both qi and blood leading to poor nour-ishment and promotion in the chong and ren chan-nels, 103

insufficiency of both qi and blood leading to poor pro-motion of blood flow and nourishment of the body, 83

insufficiency of both qi and blood resulting in poor nour-ishment of the fetus, 102

insufficiency of both qi and yin fluids, 66

insufficiency of both qi and yin leading to poor nour-ishment of the chest, 34

insufficiency of both spleen and kidney yang, 49

insufficiency of heart blood, 21, 70, 193, 197

insufficiency of heart blood and spleen qi, 222

insufficiency of heart blood leading to poor filling of blood vessels, 80

insufficiency of heart blood leading to poor nour-ishment of the heart, 254

insufficiency of heart blood leading to poor nour-ishment of the heart and mind, 222-223

insufficiency of heart blood leading to poor nour-ishment of the mind, 86

insufficiency of heart qi, 190-191, 197

insufficiency of heart qi and yang leading to poor pro-motion of heart blood, 80

insufficiency of heart qi, blood, yin, or yang leading to poor nourishment or invigoration of the heart, 190

insufficiency of heart qi leading to poor promotion of heart blood, 221

insufficiency of heart qi leading to poor promotion of the mind, 53

insufficiency of heart yang, 192, 197

insufficiency of heart yang combined with insuffi-ciency of kidney yang leading to poor warmth of the body, 234

insufficiency of heart yang leading to poor promo-tion of the blood circulation, 225

insufficiency of heart yin, 193, 197

insufficiency of heart yin resulting in production of deficiency heat, 80

insufficiency of heat leading to impairment of body fluids, 49

insufficiency of kidney essence, 21-22, 31, 214

insufficiency of kidney essence and blood, 21

insufficiency of kidney essence and qi leading to poor development, 35

insufficiency of kidney essence and qi leading to poor promotion and nourishment of hearing, 84

insufficiency of kidney essence leading to poor devel-opment, 34-35, 37

insufficiency of kidney essence leading to poor filling of sea of marrow, 74, 79

insufficiency of kidney essence leading to poor nour-ishment and promotion of the body and mind, 212

insufficiency of kidney leading to poor nourishment of the lumbar area, 77

insufficiency of kidney qi, 17, 215

insufficiency of kidney qi and yin leading to dys-function in water metabolism, 88

insufficiency of kidney qi causing failure to grasp lung qi, 35

insufficiency of kidney qi failing to grasp qi in res-piration., 215

insufficiency of kidney qi leading to an upsurge of cold water, 91

insufficiency of kidney qi leading to dysfunction in opening and closing of the bladder, 94-96

insufficiency of kidney qi leading to lack of con-solidation in the chong and ren channels, 102-103

insufficiency of kidney qi leading to loss of control of the anus, 94

insufficiency of kidney qi leading to poor consoli-dation, 254

insufficiency of kidney qi leading to poor consoli-dation, 98

insufficiency of kidney qi leading to poor consoli-dation of sperm, 97

insufficiency of kidney qi leading to poor promo-tion and nourishment of the spine, 37

insufficiency of kidney qi leading to poor promo-tion of hearing, 84

insufficiency of kidney-spleen yang leading to life gate fire failing to generate earth (spleen), 93

insufficiency of kidney yang, 213, 217

insufficiency of kidney yang leading to poor closing and opening of the bladder, 225

insufficiency of kidney yang leading to poor warmth, 97

insufficiency of kidney yang leading to poor warmth of skeleton, 225

insufficiency of kidney yang leading to poor warmth of the bladder, 217 insufficiency of kidney yang leading to the life gate fire failing to generate spleen-earth, 258

insufficiency of kidney yang qi leading to dysfunc-tion in opening and closing of the bladder, 95

insufficiency of kidney yin, 214

insufficiency of kidney yin leading to poor nour-ishment of tendons and bones, 256

insufficiency of kidney yin leading to poor nour-ishment of the body and production of defi-ciency heat, 223

insufficiency of kidney yin leading to poor nour-ishment of the mind, 256

insufficiency of kidney yin leading to weakening of the lower body, 224

insufficiency of kidney yin producing deficiency fire flaring upward and injuring blood vessels, 32

insufficiency of kidney yin (water) in the lower body, 70, 86

insufficiency of liver and kidney yin leading to poor nourishment, 99

insufficiency of liver and kidney yin leading to rising of liver yang, 34

insufficiency of liver blood, 203, 209

insufficiency of liver blood leading to poor nour-ishment of the eyes, 84, 202, 222

insufficiency of liver blood leading to poor nour-ishment of the eyes, tendons, and vessels, 254

insufficiency of liver blood leading to poor nour-ishment of the tissues and organs related to the liver, 203

insufficiency of liver-kidney yin causing stirring of defi-ciency fire, 85

insufficiency of liver yin, 204, 209

insufficiency of liver yin leading to poor nourish-ment, 256

insufficiency of liver yin leading to poor nourish-ment of the body and production of deficiency heat, 223

insufficiency of liver yin leading to the production of deficiency heat, 203

insufficiency of lung and kidney qi leading to in-ability to grasp qi, 55

insufficiency of lung and kidney yin, 57

insufficiency of lung and kidney yin leading to poor nourishment of the throat, 52

insufficiency of lung and kidney yin leading to poor nourishment of voice, 57

insufficiency of lung and kidney yin leading to pro-duction of deficiency fire, 123

insufficiency of lung and kidney yin producing defi-ciency fire flaring upward, 32

insufficiency of lung-kidney qi and yin leading to dys-function of the bladder in opening and clos-ing, 95

insufficiency of lung qi leading to poor dispersing func-tion of the lung, 253

insufficiency of lung qi leading to poor promotion of breathing, 54-55, 222

insufficiency of lung qi leading to poor promotion of respiration and voice, 221

insufficiency of lung qi leading to poor promotion of sound production, 254

insufficiency of lung qi leading to poor promotion of sound production, 56

insufficiency of lung qi leading to poor promotion of voice, 51, 56-57

insufficiency of lung yin and kidney yin, 223

insufficiency of lung yin leading to flaring of defi-ciency fire, 55

insufficiency of lung yin leading to upward flaring of deficiency fire, 75

insufficiency of pectoral qi leading to inability to sup-port speaking and breathing, 170

insufficiency of qi, 17

insufficiency of qi and blood, 18, 20

insufficiency of qi and blood leading to poor filling of blood vessels, 50

insufficiency of qi and blood leading to poor nourish-ment, 50

insufficiency of qi and blood leading to poor nourish-ment of the brain, 79

insufficiency of qi and blood leading to poor nour-ishment of the chong and ren channels, 100

insufficiency of qi, blood, and body fluids leading to poor moistening and promotion of defeca-tion, 92

insufficiency of qi, blood, essence, and marrow leading to poor nourishment, 72

insufficiency of qi, blood, yin, or yang leading to poor nourishment or promotion, 72, 77

insufficiency of qi, blood, yin, or yang leading to poor promotion and nourishment of sound pro-duction, 52

insufficiency of qi leading to hypofunction of the inter-nal organs, 219

insufficiency of qi leading to poor promotion of blood flow, 48

insufficiency of qi leading to poor tightening of muscu-lar interstices, 68

insufficiency of small intestine yang, 199

insufficiency of spleen and kidney qi leading to poor consolidation of the chong and ren chan-nels, 99

insufficiency of spleen and kidney yang, 39

insufficiency of spleen and stomach qi leading to poor promotion of sound production, 60

insufficiency of spleen and stomach yang leading to poor warmth and digestive promotion, 58

insufficiency of spleen-kidney yang leading to poor consolidation of the chong and ren channels, 101

insufficiency of spleen qi causing failure to keep blood circulating inside the blood vessels, 32, 98

insufficiency of spleen qi leading to dysfunction in transformation, 92

insufficiency of spleen qi leading to dysfunction of the spleen in transportation and transformation, 253

insufficiency of spleen qi leading to failure of the spleen to transport damp, 82

insufficiency of spleen qi leading to poor consolida-tion of heart fluids (sweats), 70

insufficiency of spleen qi leading to poor promotion of digestion, 89

insufficiency of spleen qi leading to poor promotion of lucid yang, 66

insufficiency of spleen qi leading to poor promotion of stomach qi, 102

Diagnosis in Traditional Chinese Medicine

insufficiency of spleen qi leading to poor transpor-tation and transformation of foodstuff and damp, 221, 223

insufficiency of spleen qi resulting in dysfunction in keeping the blood within the vessels, 104

insufficiency of spleen yang leading to dysfunction in transportation and transformation, 258

insufficiency of spleen yang leading to poor trans-portation and transformation, 225

insufficiency of spleen yang leading to poor trans-portation of body fluids, 49

insufficiency of stomach and spleen qi leading to poor promotion of digestion, 91

insufficiency of stomach qi leading to poor promo-tion of sound production, 58-59

insufficiency of stomach qi leading to poor promo-tion of voice, 57

insufficiency of stomach yang leading to poor warmth of the stomach, 76

insufficiency of stomach yin leading to poor nour-ishment of the stomach and stirring of defi-ciency fire, 90

insufficiency of stomach yin leading to production of deficiency fire, 76

insufficiency of the kidney leading to stirring of ministe-rial fire, 256

insufficiency of vital qi, 42-43, 55

insufficiency of vital qi leading to poor promotion of circulation of qi and blood, 142

insufficiency of vital qi leading to poor promotion of qi, blood, and organ function, 142

insufficiency of vital qi leading to poor promotion of the spirit, 142

insufficiency of yang and qi leading to looseness in the exterior, 142

insufficiency of yang leading to poor warmth, 219

insufficiency of yang leading to poor warmth of blood flow, 48

insufficiency of yang leading to poor warmth of the internal organs, channels, and network vessels, 72

insufficiency of yang qi, 68, 134

insufficiency of yang qi leading to poor promotion of blood circulation, 137, 142

insufficiency of yang qi leading to poor promotion of the flow of qi and blood, 73

insufficiency of yang qi leading to poor warmth and promotion of qi and blood, 124

insufficiency of yang qi leading to poor warmth of the body, 122, 137

insufficiency of yang qi leading to poor warmth of the limbs, 123

insufficiency of yang qi leading to the production of internal cold, 47

insufficiency of yang qi producing internal cold, 130

insufficiency of yin and blood, 19

insufficiency of yin fluids, 134

insufficiency of yin fluids giving rise to heat and com-pressing fluids outward, 70

insufficiency of yin fluids leading to poor nourish-ment, 142

insufficiency of yin fluids leading to production of defi-ciency heat, 218

insufficiency of yin fluids producing deficiency fire burning the network vessels, 72

insufficiency of yin fluids producing deficiency heat, 123

insufficiency of yin fluids producing deficiency heat, then steaming outward, 139

insufficiency of yin fluids producing internal heat, 130

insufficiency of yin fluids producing upward stir-ring of deficiency heat, 139

insufficiency of yin producing deficiency heat and steaming sweat outward, 142

interior cold pattern, 68, 130, 151, 155, 176

interior deficiency pattern, 130, 176

interior fire pattern, 157

interior heat pattern, 47, 67, 151

interior pattern, 13, 42, 46, 113, 115, 122, 129

interior wind pattern, 25

internal heat dispersing outward, 232

internal heat pressing body fluids outward, 240

internal heat promoting blood circulation, 240

internal heat stirring and forcing body fluids out-ward, 67

internal injury due to dysfunction of the internal organs, 46

internal pathogens accumulating in the interior of the body, 144

intolerance to cold, 63

introversion, 197

invasion of cold damp disturbing qi and blood flow, 77

invasion of external cold leading to tightness of the mus-cular interstices, 64

invasion of external heat leading to accumulation of wei qi in the exterior of the body, 64

invasion of external pathogens, 72

invasion of external wind cold leading to obstruc-tion of lung qi, 56

invasion of external wind leading to failure of the lung to dredge the water passages, 82

invasion of external wind leading to stagnation of qi and blood in the upper back, 73

invasion of heat at the blood level, 40

invasion of heat leading to the production of stom-ach heat, 186

invasion of the lung by dryness, 56

invasion of wind cold, 47

invasion of wind, cold, and damp leading to ob-struction of qi and blood in the channels and network ves-sels, 78

invasion of wind cold leading to tightness of the muscu-lar interstices, 104

invisible qi stagnating in the abdomen, 125

involuntary convulsions of the extremities, 209

involuntary shaking, 20

iritis, 27

irregular flow of heart qi, 195

irregular menstruation, 202

irritability, 21, 25, 27, 30-31, 50, 65, 69-70, 74-75, 80-81, 85-86, 90, 92, 97- 99, 102, 104, 134, 137, 139,

M

macules and papules, 87

madness, 190

Mai Jing (Pulse Classic), 2, 107, 109

malar flush, 52, 65, 74, 88, 133, 139, 171, 176, 193, 204, 206, 214, 218, 223, 247

malaria, 66, 136

malnutrition with strong desire to eat clay, raw rice, and other unusual things, 91

malnutrition, 38

mania, 159, 196, 231

massage, 3

massive damp retained in the body, 183

measles, 123

menopausal pattern, 254

menorrhalgia, 181

menses, heavy, 214-215, 218, 220, 222

menstruation with light-colored and thin blood, 98

menstruation, dark and scant, 99

menstruation, dark and thick with blood clots, 99

menstruation, dark red color with clots, 61

menstruation, delayed, 164-165

menstruation, delayed and scant, 203

menstruation, delayed, short, scant, and light red in color, 203

menstruation, excessive with dark-colored and thick blood, 98

menstruation, foul-smelling and of thick consis-tency, 61

menstruation, irregular, 99

menstruation, light-colored and thin, 99

menstruation, light red-colored, delayed and scant, 220, 222

menstruation, massive, 181

menstruation, obstructed, 165

menstruation, scant, 214, 218, 254

menstruation, scant and of a light color, 164

menstruation, scant with blood clots, 165

menstruation, scant with light-colored and thin vaginal blood, 98

menstruation, scant with purple-colored vaginal blood with clots, 99

mental confusion, 85, 87, 190, 196-197, 231, 243, 248

mental deficiency, 20

mental depression, 58, 76, 195, 201-202

mental disturbance, 240-241

metrorrhagia, 99, 117

middle burner pattern (yang type), 246

middle burner pattern (yin type), 247

mind, hyperactive, 86

Ming (1368-1644 C.E.), 2

miscarriage, 103, 215, 220, 222

moodiness, 102

morning sickness, 90

mouth and throat, dry, 142

mouth ulcers, 190

mouth, deviated, 30

mouth, dry, 139, 235

mouth, inability to open, 30

mouth, lips, nose, and throat, dry, 156

moxa, 3

mumps, 23

muscle twitching, 203, 207

muscular atrophy, 25, 38

muscular atrophy and flaccidity, 36

muscular constriction of the lumbar area, 37

muttering, 53, 190, 197

myasthenia gravis, 25

N

nails, pale, 164, 220, 254

nails, pale and brittle, 207

nails, pale, ridged and/or brittle, 203

nails, sallow or pale, 222

Nan Jing (Classic of Difficulties), 107, 109

nasal bleeding, 29, 173

nasal discharge, thick, 139

nasal discharge, thin, 137

nasal discharge, turbid, 29

nasal discharge, yellow, 139

nasal discharge, yellow sticky, 172

nausea and poor appetite, 85

nausea and vomiting, 136, 183, 233

nausea, 26, 81, 86, 155-156, 158-159, 163, 185-187, 189, 211, 226-227

neck and upper back rigidity, 19

neck flaccidity, 20, 34

neck stiffness, 20, 33, 37, 176, 243

necrosis and scaling of fingers or toes, 40

Nei Jing (Classic of Internal Medicine), 2, 9

nephritis, 250, 257

neurasthenia, 255

night blindness, 202-203, 207, 220, 222

night fever, 65, 256

night sweats, 27, 30, 56, 65-66, 68, 80, 85-86, 89, 134, 142, 171, 176, 187, 193, 197, 204, 206, 214, 218, 223, 235, 256-257

nocturnal emission, 79, 97, 207, 212, 214, 223-224, 256

nocturnal urination, 215, 222

noninteraction of heart and kidney, 70, 86, 224, 257

nose, runny or stuffy, 51, 132, 155

nose, runny with yellow nasal discharge, 132

nose, stuffy, 154

numbness of extremities, 20, 79, 220, 222

numbness of the body, 21, 83, 164, 203, 220, 222

numbness of the extremities and skin, 203, 207

numbness or tingling of the fingers and toes, 103

O

obesity, 159, 198, 257

obstruction at opening of the lung, 172

obstruction by calculus, 94

obstruction of blood circulation, 27, 72, 189, 195, 197

obstruction of flow of both qi and blood, 164-165, 170, 189

obstruction of heart, 192

obstruction of heart vessels leading to poor nour-ishment of the heart, 81

obstruction of lung qi in the chest, 170

pathogenic damp which is sticky causing stagnating heat in the interior of the body, 65
pathogenic dryness damaging body fluids, 157
pathogenic factors accumulating in the body, 122
pathogenic factors attacking the stomach and stag-nating in the stomach leading to reversal of stomach qi, 58-59
pathogenic factors leading to excitement of the mind, 53
pathogenic factors neither external nor internal, 5
pathogenic heat accumulating in the lower abdomen with blood stasis, 231
pathogenic heat impairing the body fluids, leading to poor moisture of the intestinal tract, 246
pathogenic heat remaining in the exterior of the body, 132
pathogenic heat restricted by damp andunable to steam outward, 247
pathogenic heat restricting yang qi inside, leading to an inability to warm the limbs, 246
pathogenic heat steaming outward and upward, 246
pathogenic heat stirring upward and affecting the mind, 246
pathogenic wind cold attacking the exterior of the body, 229
pathogenic wind, cold, summerheat, dryness, fire, toxins or insect bites attacking the body, caus-ing vital qi to rise against invading pathogens, 144
pathogens as well as the illness itself presenting yang properties, 130
pathogens as well as the illness itself presenting yin properties, 130
pathogens attacking the half exterior-half interior area of the body, 66
pathogens attacking the jue yin channel, 74
pathogens attacking the lung leading to stagnation of lung qi, 51
pathogens attacking the shao yang channel, 74
pathogens attacking the stomach leading to reversal of stomach qi, 57
pathogens attacking the tai yang channel, 74
pathogens attacking the yang ming channel, 74
pathogens entering and residing in the depths of the body, 122
pathogens entering the half exterior-half interior area of the body, 66
pathogens entering the shao yang channel leading to obstruction of qi in the channel, 136
pathogens fighting to break down the body's resis-tance at the half interior-half exterior point of the body, 76, 233
pathogens invading and staying on the surface of the body, 122
pathogens staying in the exterior of the body lead-ing to dysfunction of the lung in dispersing and precipitat-ing, 245
pathogens, external, 131
perifocal inflammation, 256
petechia, 29, 32, 99, 164, 241
phlegm accumulating in localized area, 159
phlegm accumulating in the chest, 17

phlegm accumulating in the heart vessel, 195
phlegm accumulation leading to blood stasis, 198
phlegm accumulation pattern, 159, 175, 194, 198
phlegm combined with qi accumulating in the neck, 203
phlegm combined with qi accumulating in the throat, 203
phlegm damp disturbing the chest leading to stagna-tion of lung qi, 80
phlegm damp disturbing the spleen leading to fail-ure of lucid yang to rise, 87
phlegm damp pattern, 47, 54, 87
phlegm fire accumulating in the body, 196
phlegm fire flaring upward, 196
phlegm fire pattern, 119
phlegm fire stirring the mind, 159
phlegm fire stirring upward, 210
phlegm fluids accumulating in the chest leading reversal of lung qi, 55
phlegm fluids pattern, 5, 16-17, 20, 55, 75, 89, 117, 122
phlegm fluids retained in the chest and hypochon-drium, 160
phlegm fluids retained in the chest and hypochon-drium leading to the stagnation of qi and blood, 160
phlegm fluids retained in the head, 28
phlegm fluids retained in the hypochondrium, 75
phlegm fluids retained in the lung, 160
phlegm fluids retained in the lung leading to rever-sal of lung qi, 160, 174
phlegm fluids retained in the pericardium, 160
phlegm fluids retained in the stomach, 160
phlegm fluids retained in the stomach, 89
phlegm fluids retained in the stomach and large intestine leading to reversal of stomach qi, 160
phlegm fluids retention, 124
phlegm heat accumulating in the lung leading to reversal of lung qi, 54
phlegm heat pattern, 46, 119, 125
phlegm or phlegm fluids accumulating in the chest and disturbing the flow of lung qi, 55
phlegm pattern, 5, 17, 52, 55, 79-80, 102, 117, 120
phlegm pattern combined with invasion of external pathogens, 119
phlegm retained in the chest, 55
phlegm retained in the middle burner leading to reversal of stomach qi, 159
phlegm stagnating in the lung, 175
photophobia, 85
Pi Shu (BL-20), 126
pigeon breast, 35
plague, 158
pleurisy, 75
plum pit sensation in throat, 159
pneumonia, 253
poisoning due to snake and insect venom, 158
poisoning leading to stagnation of qi and blood, 30
polydipsia, 66, 95
polyphagia, 95
polyuria, 66, 88
poor circulation of heart blood leading to poor nour-ishment of the heart, 195

poor closure of the eyelids during deep sleep, 25
poor concentration, 193, 197, 222-223
poor consolidation, 215
poor consolidation leading to disharmony between ying
and wei levels, 230
poor consolidation of semen, 215
poor consolidation of the exterior of the body, 162, 171
poor consolidation of the fetus, 215
poor consolidation of the large intestine, 178, 215
poor consolidation of the muscular interstices, 134
poor consolidation of the surface of the body, 191
poor consolidation of the thoroughfare and control-ling
channels, 215
poor consolidation of urine, 216
poor control of yin fluid leading to yang qi floating
away, 147
poor filling of the blood vessels, 164, 193, 207, 247
poor filling of the reservoir of the marrow leading to
poor nourishment of the brain, 212
poor filling of the thoroughfare and controlling channels,
202-203, 214, 220, 222
poor generation of qi and blood, 21-22
poor invigoration of the mind, 234
poor invigoration of the physical body and the vital-ity,
171, 180-181, 191
poor lifting of lucid yang, 25
poor lubrication of the intestinal tract, 134, 179, 187
poor moistening of the lips, 30
poor moistening of the mouth, 134
poor moistening of the mouth and throat, 187
poor moistening of the mouth and tongue, 179
poor nourishment and filling of the blood vessels, 215
poor nourishment of blood in its upward circulation, 171
poor nourishment of qi and blood, 181
poor nourishment of the body, 203, 207
poor nourishment of the body and extremities, 164
poor nourishment of the brain, 164
poor nourishment of the ear, 28
poor nourishment of the eyes, 27, 207
poor nourishment of the face, 164
poor nourishment of the face and the tongue, 191
poor nourishment of the gums, 32
poor nourishment of the hair, 21
poor nourishment of the hair and teeth, 214
poor nourishment of the head, 20, 204, 206
poor nourishment of the heart, 193-194
poor nourishment of the heart and spirit, 164, 220
poor nourishment of the heart leading to dysfunc-tion in
governing the blood and mind, 218
poor nourishment of the kidney leading to dysfunc-tion
in governing reproduction and stirring up ministerial fire, 218
poor nourishment of the limbs, 18, 38
poor nourishment of the lips, 30
poor nourishment of the lips and tongue, 164
poor nourishment of the liver channel, 204
poor nourishment of the liver leading to dysfunction in
spreading and precipitating, 218
poor nourishment of the lumbar region and the limbs,
205, 214

poor nourishment of the lung leading to dysfunction in
dispersing and precipitating, 218
poor nourishment of the mind leading to instability of
vital qi, 193
poor nourishment of the muscles and tendons, 19
poor nourishment of the opening of the liver, 203-204,
206
poor nourishment of the opening of the lung, 171, 173
poor nourishment of the skeleton and brain, 214
poor nourishment of the skin, 165
poor nourishment of the spleen leading to dysfunc-tion
in transporting and transforming, 218
poor nourishment of the stomach in storing food and
digesting, 186
poor nourishment of the teeth, 31
poor nourishment of the tendons and muscles, 206
poor nourishment of the tendons, nails, and eyes, 220
poor nourishment of the thoroughfare and control-ling
channels, 215
poor nourishment of the trunk and limbs, 171
poor physical and mental development, 214
poor production of blood and poor filling of the vessels,
182
poor production of blood and poor nourishment upward,
182
poor promotion and filling of blood circulation, 215
poor promotion and tonification of the brain, 162
poor promotion of blood circulation, 162, 180, 191, 192,
213, 216-217, 234, 247
poor promotion of blood circulation or dysfunction in
removing damp, 134
poor promotion of body resistance, 29
poor promotion of breathing, 17
poor promotion of intestinal qi, 234
poor promotion of lucid yang qi leading to a poor hold
on the internal organs, 181
poor promotion of qi and blood circulation to nour-ish
the body, 215-216
poor promotion of qi circulating in the vessels, 182
poor promotion of qi flow in the chest, 191
poor promotion of the blood vessels, 135
poor promotion of the heart vessel, 171
poor promotion of yang qi, 258
poor provision of qi and blood, 20
poor regulation of stomach qi, 235
poor restoration and consolidation of the urinary system,
258
poor source of menstrual blood, 164
poor source of nutritive substances leading to poor nourishment of the limbs and body, 180
poor splenic transportation and transformation func-tion,
234
poor support of the splenic functions of transporta-tion
and transformation, 202
poor transformation of qi and blood, 180-181
poor transportation and transformation of body fluids,
192
poor transportation by the spleen, 182
poor transportation of water damp, 39
poor upward nourishment of the head and face, 193

poor warming of the uterus for women, 213
poor warmth and poor circulation of qi and blood, 208
poor warmth due to yang deficiency, 258
poor warmth leading to lack of consolidation of the
    bladder, 217
poor warmth of qi and blood leading to an obstruc-tion
    in their circulation, 192
poor warmth of the abdomen, 182, 199, 234
poor warmth of the body, 134, 192, 196, 217, 234
poor warmth of the body and limbs, 147, 178, 182, 213
poor warmth of the large intestine, 178
poor warmth of the stomach, 187
postpartum disorders, 103
postpartum fever, 104
postures, forced, 17
preference for solitude, 190
pregnancy, 35
premature ejaculation, 97, 212-213, 215, 219
prevalence of pathogenic factors with strong vital qi, 130
prolapse of internal organs, 17, 181, 184, 219, 223
prolapse of the eyelids, 25
prolapse of the rectum, 249
prolapse of the uterus, rectum, stomach, and kid-neys,
    162
prolapse of the viscera, 162
prosperity of yang, disorders occurring in the qi level, 72
prosperity of yin, disorders occurring in the blood level,
    72
proteinuria, 250
pruritus of the vulva, 207
pulmonary abscess, 61, 75
pulmonary emphysema, 35, 252-253
pulmonary heart disease, 252-253
pulmonary infections, 29
pulmonary tuberculosis, 256
pulse, bird-pecking, 119
pulse, bubble-rising, 118
pulse, choppy, 81, 89, 99-100, 104, 113, 117, 165-166,
    189, 197, 225
pulse, deep, 112, 115, 232
pulse, deep choppy, 119, 231
pulse, deep forceless, 257
pulse, deep indistinct, 213, 215
pulse, deep moderate, 119
pulse, deep rolling, 120
pulse, deep-seated, 115
pulse, deep slow, 80, 92, 100, 119-120, 135, 196, 198-
    199, 219, 234
pulse, deep slow strong, 64
pulse, deep slow weak, 64
pulse, deep slow with forceful beat, 155, 232, 246
pulse, deep slow with forceless beat, 178, 182, 187
pulse, deep tense, 174, 176, 188, 201
pulse, deep thin, 119, 215, 257-258
pulse, deep thin choppy, 253
pulse, deep thin knotted, 252
pulse, deep thin rapid, 253
pulse, deep weak, 217, 257
pulse, deep wiry, 119
pulse, distinct, 166

pulse, distinctive or deep and slow with forceless beat-
    ing, 135
pulse, distinct with forceless beating, 142
pulse, feeble, 80, 87, 116
pulse, firm, 117
pulse, fish-swimming, 118
pulse, flicking-stone, 118
pulse, floating, 21, 3, 51, 55-56, 82, 104, 112, 114, 154,
    156, 160, 175, 251
pulse, floating moderate, 67, 119, 154
pulse, floating rapid, 64, 67, 73, 119-120, 132, 176, 242,
    245
pulse, floating rapid with forceless beat, 148, 247
pulse, floating rolling, 119-120
pulse, floating tense, 29, 64, 68, 115, 119, 132, 176, 230
pulse, floating wiry, 251
pulse, flooding, 67, 88, 113, 116, 232, 240
pulse, flooding at the cun (inch) position on both sides,
    245
pulse, flooding rapid, 119, 134, 242
pulse, flooding rapid with forceless beating, 146
pulse, forceful rapid, 70
pulse, flooding rolling rapid, 157, 240
pulse, hollow, 115
pulse, hurried, 29, 113, 118
pulse, indistinct, 69, 116, 147-148, 192
pulse, intermittent, 113, 118, 191-192, 219
pulse, knotted, 113, 118, 191-192, 219231
pulse, long, 113, 116
pulse, moderate, 113, 115, 120
pulse, moderate floating, 230
pulse, moving, 117
pulse, rapid, 17, 21, 40, 61, 69, 98, 99, 104, 113, 115,
    120, 139, 165-166, 188, 194, 200
pulse, rapid floating, 157, 172-173, 231, 239
pulse, rapid soggy, 185
pulse, rapid thin, 85, 90
pulse, rapid with forceful beat, 174
pulse, rapid with forceless beat, 155
pulse, replete, 113
pulse, replete with forceful beating, 144
pulse, rolling, 17, 31, 81, 90, 113, 117, 159, 175-176,
    189, 195, 198
pulse, rolling rapid, 92, 119, 196, 217
pulse, rolling with forceful beat, 158
pulse, roof-leaking, 119
pulse, rope-untying, 119
pulse, scattered, 115
pulse, short, 113, 116
pulse, shrimp-darting, 118
pulse, slow, 113, 115, 120, 137, 234
pulse, soft, 87-88, 117, 155, 185
pulse, soft slow, 227
pulse, soggy rapid, 178, 184, 247
pulse, soggy slow, 183, 185
pulse, swift, 115, 148
pulse, tense, 68, 117, 120
pulse, tense floating, 172
pulse, thin, 21, 32, 74, 80, 84, 98, 100, 116, 164, 193,
    220, 222, 254-255

rectal collapse following defecation, 94
redness and swelling of the gums, 251
redness, swelling, and sensation of heat, 78
restlessness of the mind, 194
restlessness, 50, 53, 87, 253, 257
restraint of wei qi leading to an obstruction of qi and
    blood circulation, 231
restriction of yang qi by internal cold leading to poor
    promotion of sweating, 68
retardation, 105
retention of body fluids, 16, 125, 183
retention of body fluids in the skin and limbs, 170
retention of body fluids leading to production of phlegm,
    170
retention of body fluids leading to water qi attack-ing the
    heart, 81
retention of urine, 94, 212-213, 219
reversal of lung qi, 17, 245
reversal of qi from the chong vessel leading to re-versal
    of stomach qi, 90
reversal of stomach qi, 57, 183, 187, 189, 200, 233
reversal pattern, 115
reverting liver qi pattern, 163
reverting lung qi pattern, 163
reverting stomach qi pattern, 163
rhinorrhea, 29
Ri Yue (GB-24), 126
rickets, 20
rise of deficiency fire, 16
rise of liver fire causing reversal of lung qi., 225
rising of deficiency fire, 134
rising of liver fire leading to qi and blood rushing up,
    226
rising of liver wind, 18, 42
running piglet qi, 235
runny nose, 172

S

saliva, expectoration of copious thin clear, 160
saliva, expectoration of sticky, 159
saliva, thin, 137
salty taste, 91
scleritis, 25
scrofula, 159
scrotum, pain radiating to the lower abdomen, 208
scrotum, swelling, pain, and distension, 207
secretions and excretions heavy or foul-smelling, 144
seminal emission, 97, 220, 222
senility, 31, 214
separation of yin fluids and yang qi, 235
seven emotions, 5
sexual activity, 39
sexual function, hyperactive, 214, 218
Shang Han Za Bing Lun (On Cold Damage and Miscel-
    laneous Diseases), 2
shao yang pattern, 66, 76, 136, 233
shao yin cold pattern, 234
shao yin heat pattern, 235
Shen Men (HT-7), 110
Shen Shu (BL-23), 126

Shi Wen (Ten Questions/ (Ten Aspects to Interro-gate in
    Verse), 2
shingles, 207
shortness of breath, 17, 29, 54-55, 57, 69, 80, 82, 85,
    142, 147, 155, 162, 170, 184, 190-191, 197, 198,
    216, 219, 252-254
shouting in a high voice, 190
sighing, 51, 60, 75, 81, 163, 165, 201, 250
sighing, frequent, 202, 226, 258-259
simultaneous transmission along two or three chan-nels,
    236
sinking of spleen qi pattern, 94
sinusitis, 29, 60
six environmental phenomena, 5
skin and sclera bright yellow, 75
skin and whites of eyes bright yellow, 184
skin dry without luster, 16
skin lesion, 40
skin lesions in the pudendal region, 207
skin lesions with itching, 154
skin rashes, 154
skin rashes with itching, 156
skin, bruises, 157
skin, dry, possibly chapped, 156
skin, scaly and dry, 165
sleepiness, 87
small intestine cold accumulation pattern, 201
small intestine deficiency cold pattern, 199
small intestine excess heat pattern, 200
small intestine qi obstruction pattern, 200
sneezing, 132, 154
snoring, 52
snoring due to poor sleeping position, 52
snoring due to overweight, 52
snoring with chronic nasal disorders, 52
snoring with loss of consciousness, 52
somnolence, 142, 253-254
sore throat, 61, 64, 67, 73, 132, 151, 154, 157, 172, 239,
    242, 245
soreness and discomfort of the whole body, 132
soreness and flaccidity of the loin and knees, 86
soreness and flaccidity of the lumbar area, 77
soreness and flaccidity of the lumbar area and knees, 17,
    85, 95, 205, 209
soreness and flaccidity of the lumbar area and limbs, 70,
    74
soreness and pain of the lumbar area and limbs, 257
soreness and pain of the whole body, 156
soreness and weakness in the loin and knees, 93
soreness and weakness of the lumbar area and knees, 96-
    97, 100, 160, 214-216, 218, 220, 222-225, 256
soreness and weakness of the lumbar region, 215
soreness of the lumbar area, 78-79
soreness of the lumbar area and knees, 99
sores in the mouth, 188
sores of the mouth and the tongue, 194, 200
sores on tongue body and in the mouth, 224
sores, 158
sour taste, 91
spasms of the limbs, 20, 31, 33, 37, 50

spasms of the muscles, 78
speaking in low voice, 142
speaking that consumes qi, 171
speech that is weak, low, and incoherent, 53
speech, deranged, 53
speech, deranged with a sharp loud voice, 53
speech, difficult 205
speech, no desire for, 137, 162, 170-171, 184
spermatorrhea, 97, 212-213, 215
spitting, 55
splashing sound in the abdomen, 160
splashing sound in the upper abdomen, 89
spleen and stomach cold damp, 227
spleen deficiency combined with liver qi stagnation, 119
spleen deficiency–damp accumulation pattern, 119
spleen deficiency–food stagnation pattern, 158
spleen deficiency leading to the production of cold damp ,234
spleen deficiency pattern, 81-82, 91
spleen failing to contain blood inside the vessels, 184
spleen qi deficiency, 25, 219
spleen qi deficiency failing to keep blood circulat-ing in the vessels, 29, 167
spleen qi deficiency leading to dysfunction of the spleen in transporting and transforming damp, leading to water retention, 160
spleen qi deficiency leading to failure of lucid yang to rise, 87
spleen qi deficiency leading to poor promotion of diges-tion, 255
spleen qi deficiency leading to poor promotion of the spirit, 255
spleen qi deficiency leading to poor transportation and transformation of foodstuff, 158
spleen qi deficiency leading to sinking of lucid yang, 85
spleen qi deficiency pattern, 14, 20-21, 25, 29, 32, 66, 87, 89, 92, 98, 102, 104, 180-182, 184
spleen qi exhaustion pattern, 119
spleen qi fall pattern, 184, 249
spleen qi-kidney qi deficiency pattern, 25, 99
spleen qi stagnating in the middle burner leading to poor digestion, 180
spleen yang deficiency pattern, 49, 182, 219
spleen yang-kidney yang deficiency pattern, 22, 93, 101, 225
spleen yang qi deficiency pattern, 160
spleen yin deficiency pattern, 218
spleen-stomach cold damp pattern, 26
spleen-stomach damp heat pattern, 61, 91, 93
spleen-stomach deficiency pattern, 35, 38
spleen-stomach qi deficiency pattern, 36, 60, 91
splenic dysfunction in transporting and transform-ing, 219
spontaneous sweating, 80, 142, 184, 191, 197-198, 219-221, 252
sputum with pus and blood, 61
sputum with wheezing sound from the throat, 144
sputum, bloody, 57, 171
sputum, clear thin white, 172
sputum, copious and easily expectorated, 175-176

sputum, foamy, 57
sputum, profuse, 55-56, 80
sputum, profuse purulent or bloody, 75
sputum, profuse thick yellow, 56
sputum, scant sticky with difficult expectoration, 171, 176
sputum, sticky scant yellow, 172
sputum, sticky yellow, 173
sputum, thick, 139
sputum, thin, 137
sputum, thin clear, 171, 221-222
sputum, thin white, 56, 174, 219, 252
sputum, white, 137
sputum, yellow, 139
stagnant blood accumulating in the channels and net-work vessels, 69
stagnated blood circulation, 198
stagnated blood excreted with stools, 231
stagnated blood obstructing the blood vessels caus-ing bleeding, 166
stagnated food transforming into heat, 61
stagnated liver qi accumulating in the chong and ren channels, 73
stagnated liver qi attacking the spleen leading to dys-function in transformation and transporta-tion, 93
stagnated liver qi attacking the stomach leading to rever-sal of stomach qi, 59, 235
stagnated liver qi producing internal heat compli-cated by an attack of wind heat, 35
stagnated liver qi stirring upward, 60
stagnated qi accumulating in the neck, 33
stagnation of blood and qi leading to obstruction, 73
stagnation of blood and qi occurring in the heart vessel, 80
stagnation of blood in the uterus, 104
stagnation of wei qi occurring on the surface of the body, 239
stagnation of food producing heat, 46, 58
stagnation of gallbladder qi, 137, 210
stagnation of gallbladder qi leading to disturbance of stomach qi, 136
stagnation of gallbladder qi leading to reversal of stom-ach qi, 233
stagnation of heart blood or lung qi, 34
stagnation of large intestine qi, 177
stagnation of liver qi, 259
stagnation of liver qi and reversal of stomach qi, 226
stagnation of liver qi attacking the spleen, 259
stagnation of liver qi caused by mental depression, 75
stagnation of liver qi leading to blood stasis, 202
stagnation of liver qi leading to obstruction of blood circulation, 35
stagnation of liver qi transversely attacking the stomach, 76, 91
stagnation of lung qi, 175
stagnation of lung qi leading to poor promotion of blood flow, 30
stagnation of phlegm damp leading to stirring up of the mind, 54
stagnation of qi along the shao yin channel, 233

tongue, red with thin coating, 176
tongue, red with thin greasy coating, 250
tongue, red with white coating, 257
tongue, red with yellow coating, 17, 48, 59, 90, 174,
    188, 194, 200, 204, 206, 209, 240
tongue, red with yellow dry coating, 134, 209, 232, 246
tongue, red with yellow greasy coating, 184-185, 207,
    247
tongue, sallow or pale, 222
tongue, scarlet stiff, 48
tongue, stiff, 49
tongue, stiff with difficulty speaking, 246
tongue, stiff with dry coating, 49
tongue, tender moist, 49
tongue, thick tender, 142
tongue, thin dark, 49
tongue, thin pale, 49
tongue, tight puffy with thick yellow coating, 144
tongue, tremors and stiffness, 50
tongue, with tooth marks, 89
tonsillitis, 33, 61
toothache, 60, 251
toxic damp, 158
toxic heat accumulating internally and blocking yang qi
    from circulating outwards, 123
toxic heat accumulating in the lung, 61, 75
toxic heat accumulating in the throat, 35, 57, 61
toxic heat entering the heart, 49
toxic heat flaring upward and accumulating in the throat,
    33
toxic heat pattern, 27, 32-33, 40, 48-49, 57, 123
toxic heat stirring upward and accumulating in the stom-
    ach channel, 32
toxic pattern, 35
toxic wind attacking the channels and network ves-sels,
    158
toxicity leading to collapse of vital qi, 27
toxicity, 19
toxin, epidemic pathogens, 158
transmission along the channels, 236
trauma impairing blood vessels, 37
trauma impairing fetal qi, 103
tremors of the limbs, 241
tremors of the muscles, 202, 209
tremors, 19
true cold presenting with false heat pattern, 15
tubercular fibrosis, 256
tuberculosis of the bones and joints, 158
tuberculosis of the lung with cavitation, 256
tuberculosis of the lymph nodes, 123
tumors, 27, 35, 164
turbid phlegm accumulating in the body and steam-ing
    outward, 195
turbid phlegm accumulating in the heart vessel, 74
turbid phlegm accumulating in the lung leading to poor
    dispersing action of the lung, 52
turbid phlegm accumulating in the stomach leading to
    reversal of stomach qi, 102
twitching of the muscles, 202
twitching or tremors of the limbs, 247

tympany, 125

U

ulcers, 35, 158
undigested food accumulating in the intestinal tract, 93
undigested food retained in the stomach, 189
undigested food retained in the stomach producing damp
    heat, 94
undigested food stagnating in the stomach leading to
    production of heat, 91
undigested food stagnating in the stomach leading to
    reversal of stomach qi, 90
unsteadiness of collapsed vital qi, 115
unsteadiness of the mind, 196
upper abdomen discomfort, 31
upper abdomen, distension, fullness and discomfort, 158
upper burner pattern, 245-246
upsurge of kidney water causing disturbances of heart qi,
    34
upward flaring of deficiency fire, 27
upward flaring of liver fire, 25-26
upward flaring of phlegm fire, 190
upward flaring of phlegm fire affecting the mind, 190,
    196
upward flaring of toxic heat, 23
upward rushing of turbid yin, 16
upward steaming of gallbladder heat, 211
upward steaming of turbid damp, 183
upward steaming of turbid stomach qi, 251
upward stirring of deficiency fire affecting the mind, 193
upward stirring of heat, 239
upward stirring of liver wind, 19-20
upward stirring of qi and blood, 18
upward stirring of wind, 19
upward stirring of wind phlegm, 18
uremia, 61, 94
urethral tract, hot sensation of, 199
urinary incontinence, 96, 142, 253-254
urinary stones, 71, 94
urinary tract infection, 94
urination, abnormal, 258
urination with burning sensation, 95, 200
urination, difficult, 94
urination, frequent, 94, 215-217, 219-220, 222
urination, frequent at night, 257
urination, urgent and painful, 216-217
urine, acrid-smelling, 61
urine, clear, 137, 152
urine, clear and in large amounts, 95, 135
urine, dark, 70
urine, dark-colored, 174, 185, 194, 209, 211
urine, dark scant, 188, 199
urine, excessive clear, 135, 151
urine, incontinence of, 17, 30, 94, 97, 215, 220
urine, scant, 68, 95, 104, 160, 182-183, 185, 225, 250-
    251, 258
urine, scant clear, 199
urine, scant dark, 94-95, 134, 139, 151, 155, 175, 165,
    183, 200, 204, 240, 246, 253
urine, scant dry, 92, 134

wind cold attacking and accumulating in the net-work vessels, 25

wind cold attacking on the surface of the body, leading to tightness of the muscular interstices, 68

wind cold attacking the body and presenting as heat, 151

wind cold attacking the exterior of the body, 138

wind cold attacking the joints leading to stagnation of qi and blood, 78

wind cold attacking the lung, 29, 172, 176

wind cold attacking the tai yang channel leading to obstruction of qi and blood, 33

wind cold attacking upward, 23

wind cold invading and remaining in the muscular interstices, fighting with wei qi on the exterior of the body, 155

wind cold invading the network vessels leading to stagnation of qi and blood, 49

wind cold remaining in the exterior of the body, 172

wind combining with cold damp and obstructing the channels and network vessels, affecting the joints, 154

wind damp, 69

wind damp exterior pattern, 74

wind damp impediment pattern, 38

wind damp obstructing the channels and network vessels, 38

wind fire flaring upward and stirring in the orifices, 85

wind heat, 35

wind heat accumulating in the liver channel, 26

wind heat accumulating in the lung channel, 29

wind heat attacking the body, presenting as cold, 151

wind heat attacking the exterior of the body, 141

wind heat attacking the joint leading to stagnation of qi and blood, 78

wind heat attacking the liver channel and flaring upward, 25

wind heat attacking the lung, 29, 52, 172

wind heat attacking the lung and accumulating in the throat, 52

wind heat attacking the skin and producing upward flaring of fire, 38

wind heat attacking the surface of the body leading to looseness of the muscular interstices, 67

wind heat pattern, 60

wind heat remaining in the exterior of the body, 172

wind impediment pattern, 38, 78, 119, 154

wind pattern, 50, 120

wind phlegm accumulating and stirring in the mind, 30

wind phlegm accumulating internally and stirring upward, 25, 27

wind phlegm accumulating in the heart and affecting the mind, 197

wind phlegm accumulating in the network vessels, 30-31, 50

wind phlegm heat pattern, 57

wind phlegm obstructing network vessels, 18

wind phlegm obstructing the internal organs, 18

wind phlegm obstructing the tongue vessel, 205

wind phlegm or blood stasis due to trauma leading to obstruction of the channels and network vessels, 69

wind phlegm pattern, 27-28, 30, 69, 119

wind phlegm stirring upward and affecting the mind, 159

wind phlegm stirring upward and obstructing the network vessels, 23

wind remaining the exterior of the body, 175

wind rising against water in the upper body, 175

wind stroke (closed type), 30

wind stroke (open type), 30

wind stroke pattern, 17, 23, 50, 69, 83, 159

wind warm disease, 23

wind water attacking the lung, 22, 82, 160, 251

wind water attacking the lung and penetrating into the skin and interstices of the muscles, 39

wind, aversion to, 132

wu mei (fructus mume), 45

Wu Jutong, 2

Wu Li (LR-10), 110

X

Xiao Chang Shu (BL-27), 126

Y

yang collapse leading to poor promotion of blood circulation, 148

yang collapse leading to yang qi flowing outward, 148

yang deficiency combined with kidney yang deficiency, 225

yang deficiency leading to failure to control the water passage, 258

yang deficiency pattern, 14, 16, 46, 48, 57, 116, 218

yang exhaustion followed by qi collapse, 167

yang exhaustion pattern, 14, 69, 80, 114, 116, 148

yang heat rising in the upper body while yin cold accumulates in the lower body, 152

yang ming bowel excess pattern, 65

yang ming bowel pattern, 53, 70, 92, 119, 232

yang ming channel pattern, 67, 232

yang pattern, 13, 40, 72, 116, 120

yang qi deficiency in the large intestine, 178

yang qi deficiency leading to poor promotion of vitality, 137

yang qi entering the interior of the body and steaming yin fluids outward, 68

yang qi failing to go out and warm the surface of the body, caused by stagnated phlegm inside the body, 174

yang qi moving inwards during sleep, assisting deficiency heat, causing the body fluids to go out, 171

yang qi restrained in the interior of the body, failing to warm the upper abdomen, 188

yang qi restricted by excess cold, 188

yang qi restricted in the body, leading to inability to warm the body and limbs, 208

yang qi, sudden loss of, 147

yang qi unable to move outward leading to poor warmth of the body, 135

yang rising in the upper body, 205

Ye Tianshi, 2

Diagnosis in Traditional Chinese Medicine

Yi Jong Jin Jian (Golden Mirror of the Medical Tradition), 109
yin cold accumulating and obstructing qi flow, 135
yin collapse leading to poor filling of the blood vessels, 148
yin collapse leading to yin qi losing its attachment and flowing outward, 148
yin deficiency combined with yang hyperactivity, 205
yin deficiency leading to deficiency heat, 48
yin deficiency leading to poor nourishment of the lips, 30
yin deficiency pattern, 15, 17, 32, 39, 47, 49, 55, 57, 65, 68, 70, 85, 88-89, 95, 116, 119, 122, 209, 218
yin deficiency producing heat, 68
yin deficiency producing heat aided by yang qi, 65
yin exhaustion pattern, 36, 46-47, 68-69, 148
yin (fluids) deficiency in the large intestine, 179
ying level pattern, 53, 87, 89
yin pattern, 13, 50, 72, 120
Yuan (1271-1368 C.E.), 2

Z

Zhang Jingyue, 2
Zhang Men (LR-13), 126
Zhang Zhongjing, 2
Zhong Fu (LU-1), 125
Zhong Ji (CV-3), 126
Zhu Bing Yuan Hou Lun (Origins and Symptoms of Diseases, 2
Zu San Li (ST-36), 126
zygomatic region, red 256